welcoming
baby

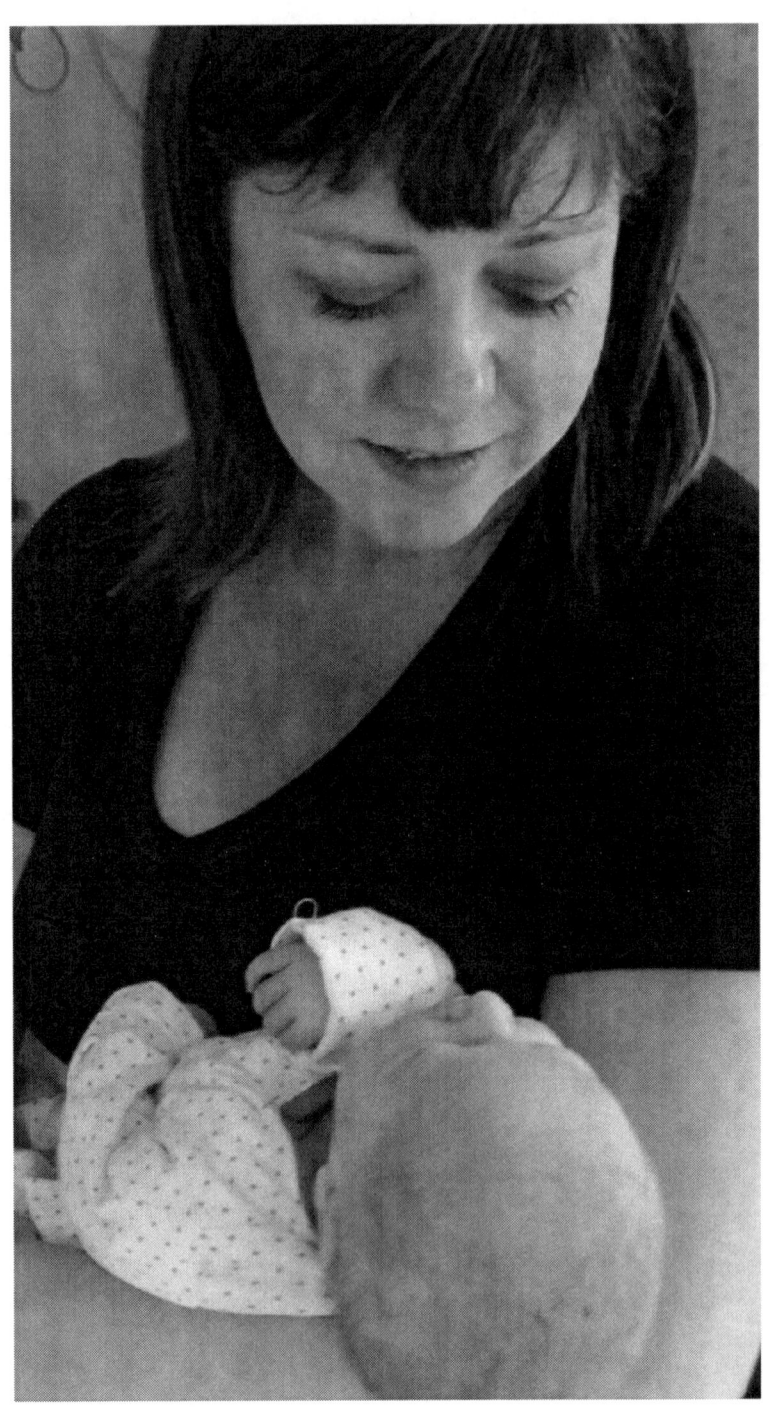

welcoming baby

— reflections on perinatal care —

Debby Gould

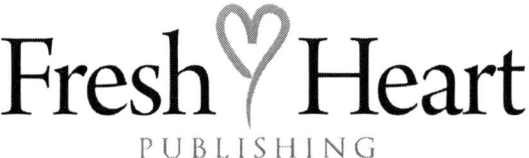
PUBLISHING

1st edition

Published in 2011 by
FRESH HEART PUBLISHING
a division of Fresh Heart Ltd
PO Box 225, Chester le Street, DH3 9BQ, United Kingdom
www.freshheartpublishing.co.uk

© Fresh Heart Publishing 2011

The moral right of Debby Gould to be identified as the author of this work has been asserted in accordance with the Copyright, Designs and Patents Act 1988.

All rights reserved. No part of this publication may be reproduced, stored in a retrieval system, or transmitted, in any form or by any means, electronic, mechanical, photocopying, recording or otherwise, without the prior permission of the publisher. Nor may this publication be circulated in any form of binding or cover other than that in which it is published and without a similar condition being imposed on the subsequent purchaser.

A CIP catalogue record for this publication is available from the British Library

ISBN: 978 1 906619 16 9

Set in Franklin Gothic Book, Eras ITC and Bradley Hand ITC
Designed and typeset by Fresh Heart Publishing
Fresh Heart Books for Better Birth series editor: Sylvie Donna
Printed in the UK by Lightning Source UK Ltd
Cover design by Fresh Heart Publishing
Cover photo by Patti Ramos, used with permission
Photos on pages ii, v, vi, x, 17, 39, 58, 68, 69, 91, 94, 106, 107 and 127
by Debby Gould, used with permission

Disclaimer

While the advice and information contained in this book are believed to be accurate and true at the time of going to press, neither the author, nor the translator, nor the publisher can accept any legal responsibility for loss, damage or injury occasioned to any person acting or refraining from action as a result of information contained. These suggestions are guidelines only and should be used alongside advice from midwives or obstetricians.

Dedication

This is for all who dare to doubt the certainty of some of our current practices around childbirth, and care enough to dream that we can reframe and refocus the how and what of midwifery. Learning to be comfortable with uncertainty is an essential skill for everyone to master in life; it is especially so for midwives. Uncertainty keeps us interested, keeps us learning, but most of all keeps us all safe and curiously passionate to continuously improve care.

For my sister, Cathy, who one insignificant day at an unspecified time, unknowingly planted an acorn deep within me to champion women, childbirth, midwives and midwifery, and without whom this book would never have been written.

With thanks to my best friend Liz Stephens, and my two sons Will and Josh, whose unconditional love and support I am blessed with. Thanks too for my publisher's skill and unending patience.

Note: This book is written predominantly for people working in an NHS England hospital unit and while many practices may be similar in some areas or across the world they may also differ widely. In addition, the experience in some midwifery-led birth centres may be different as this book focuses mainly on the hospital experience.

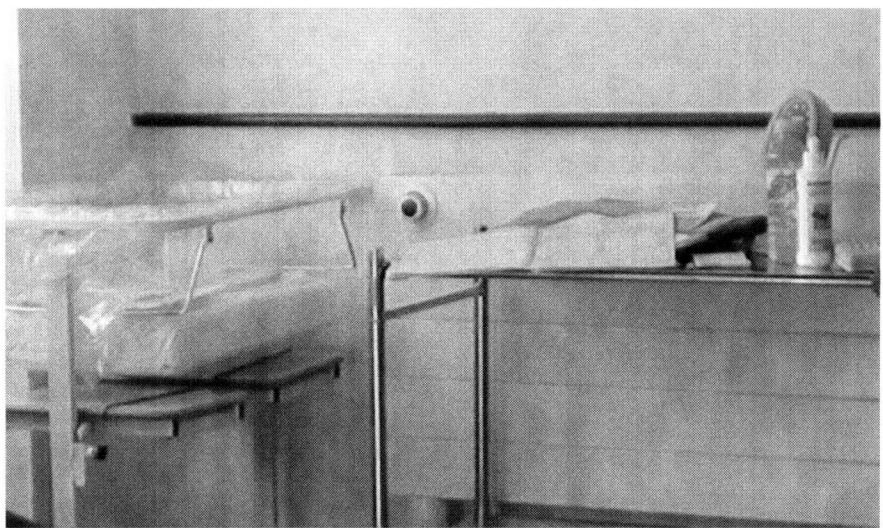

A bassinet intended for a newborn, with some day-to-day equipment nearby

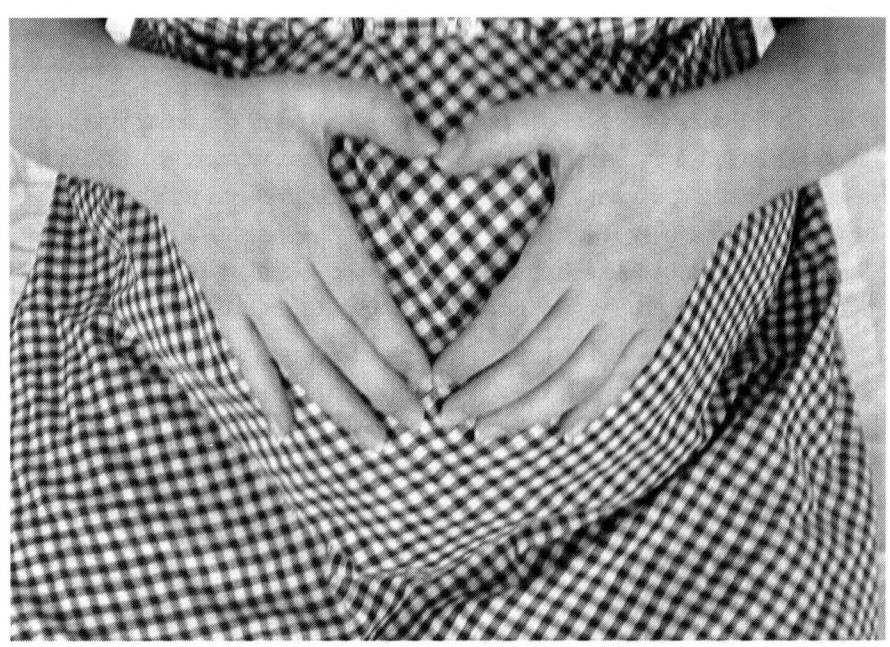
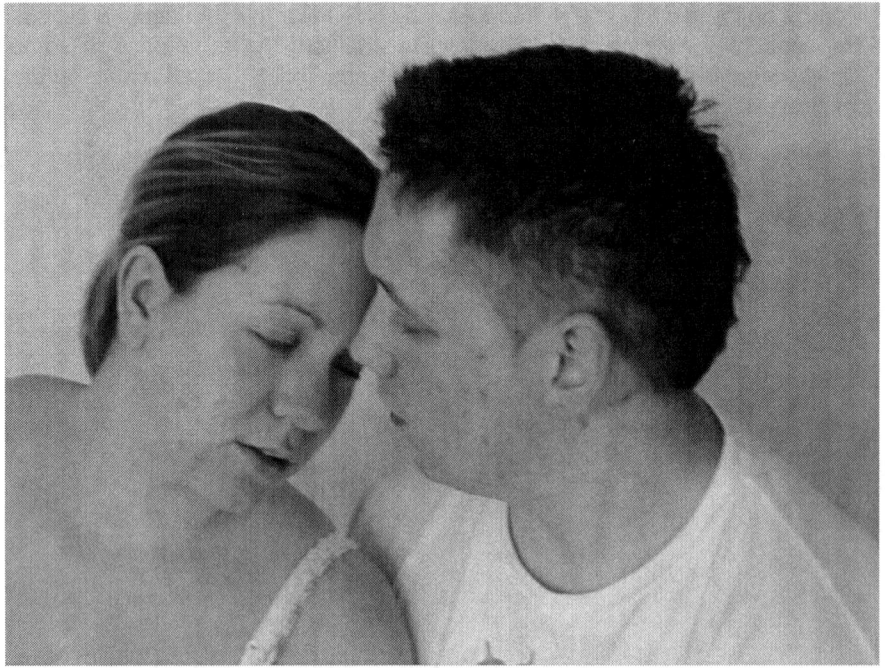

Waiting for the new baby... then labouring towards his or her arrival: a special time in a woman's life

Contents

Dedication   v

Foreword by Liz Stephens, President of the Royal College of Midwives   viii

Chapter 1:   **An unnoticed problem**   1

Chapter 2:   **The situation today**   10

Chapter 3:   **A developing outlook towards maternity care**   24

Chapter 4:   **Alienation and efficiency in postmodern institutions**   42

Chapter 5:   **The politics and power of language**   52

Chapter 6:   **Patterns of power in the delivery suite**   64

Chapter 7:   **Ritualised care in the light of the evidence**   76

Chapter 8:   **Facilitating the transition to motherhood**   96

Chapter 9:   **Mismatched perceptions in the media and real life**   110

Chapter 10:   **From conspiratorial models to an inspirational approach**   122

Chapter 11:   **Using all aspects of communication to really welcome the baby**   138

Chapter 12:   **Making a positive experience a life-enhancing one**   164

Index   182

Also available   190

About the author   192

Foreword

Twenty years on from the publication of the Winterton Report (Department of Health, 1991) Debby Gould takes a critical look at today's maternity services. The Winterton Report, which followed a pivotal enquiry in the history of our maternity services, was the report of a Health Committee that took note of the views of the users of maternity services, as well as the professionals providing those services. The findings of this enquiry then resulted in another report, *Changing Childbirth* (Department of Health, 1993); this report, which was again written by a committee of experts, supported choice, continuity and control for women and it respected the notion of midwifery-led care. When it was published it seemed to signal the dawn of a new era, when women and midwives would work together delivering a safe service that offered women respect and choice, both of which would support normal birth. Two decades later, Debby looks at the state of the maternity service today—a time when we have caesarean section rates that have been spiralling out of control, leading to a decrease in normal birth, and homebirth rates that have hardly risen, despite policy that supports this choice. She considers a service that all too often puts institutions and their policies, norms and rituals at the centre of care, rather than the women and babies who should surely be the focus. The time is right for the critical examination of maternity care which this book provides.

It is no coincidence that as maternity care has become increasingly hospitalised rates of intervention have also risen. In this book Debby Gould highlights how in the institutionalised and mechanistic model of care which is a feature of large maternity units, the emotion and love that should abound so as to welcome a new life are increasingly marginalised. At times this book makes for uncomfortable reading as Debby exposes the ways in which midwifery culture is complicit in supporting a model of care that can be disrespectful to women—and indeed babies!—and which can diminish the crucial rite of passage of childbirth in the lives of both women and their babies.

> The author has highlighted how in the institutionalised and mechanistic model of care which is a feature of large maternity units, the emotion and love that should abound so as to welcome a new life are increasingly marginalised

Debby analyses the use of language and shows how it serves to perpetuate professional dominance, detract attention from individual women and decrease their sense of ownership of the childbirth experience. She also emphasises the need for us all to critique our individual motivation and behaviours, as well as those of the institutions we work within. In addition, she draws our attention to the stark contrasts between nurturing ways of caring and the institutionalised practices and procedures that are currently the norm. Overall, she explains how, in our constant striving for safety, we have lost an element of caring and nurturing, even though safety and caring/nurturing should be interdependent, not mutually exclusive. She persuasively explains why we should be prioritising nurturing ways of caring at this pivotal time in the lives of women and their families, and not marginalising this vital aspect of care.

Focusing on practical ways forward, Debby looks at techniques used in other disciplines so as to demonstrate ways in which we can work to improve communication. She shows how these techniques can be used to help women perceive the positive aspects of labour and birth rather than the negative, even though these are not yet valued in organizations, which at times appear to value empirical knowledge above emotion and caring.

All in all, this book challenges us to look more closely at the routines and rituals of common hospital practice and it prompts us to consider whether some of them are actually damaging to the establishment of the mother-baby relationship. This relationship is fundamental to the psychological well-being of the woman and baby as well to wider family dynamics. Yet—as Debby points out—this fact seems to have got lost in the policies and procedures of our labour wards, where 'safe delivery' has become an end in itself. While safe delivery is obviously important, Debby helps us to see why the most important aspect of birth is the quality of the beginning of a new life. She shows how it should not an end in itself, separate from other concerns, but the beginning of a whole new life experience.

I believe this book is essential reading for everyone involved in maternity services because it will help us to conduct a more open debate on the nature of the service we offer women. It should help students, who are the future of the maternity service, to understand the enormous potential they have to promote good midwifery care so as to benefit both women and their families, and of course the babies to whom they give birth.

Liz Stephens, RGN, RM, BSc (Hons), PG Dip Ed, MA, MSc
President of the Royal College of Midwives

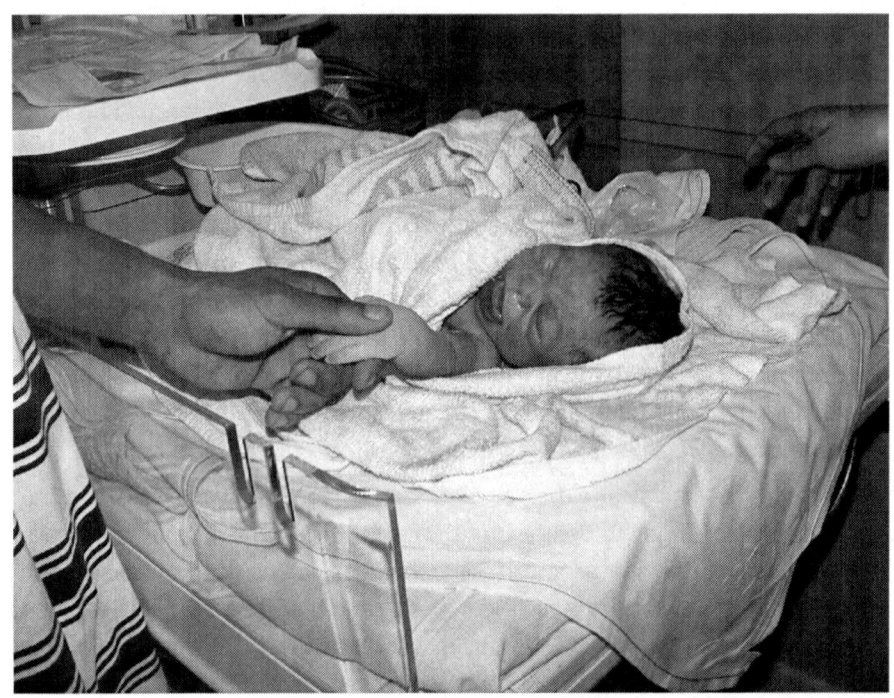

How often do we notice the emotional state of the newborn baby?

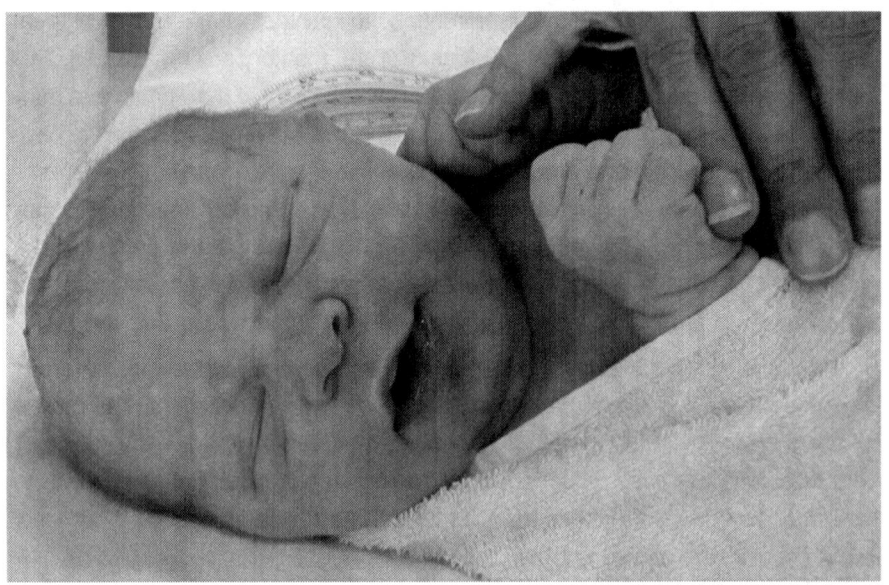

1: An unnoticed problem

"Faith and doubt both are needed—not as antagonists, but working side by side to take us around the unknown curve."

Lillian Smith (1897-1966), American novelist

THE IMPORTANCE OF THE PERINATAL PERIOD

The relationship forged between a newborn human baby and his or her family, particularly his or her mother, is as crucial as the relationship any baby mammal forms when born in the wild—if not more so. A human child is dependent on its carers for infinitely longer than all other mammals. Furthermore, the woman's (and sometimes the father's) sense of self is often defined by how she perceives herself as a mother (or he as a father). Whether it is recognised or not, this psychological co-dependency between parents and babies unites and supports all humanity and it is therefore more important than many of the physical aspects of childbirth, except for the prevention of harm.

We have all experienced the moment of our own birth. Our bodies were so full of adrenaline (because of our own fear) and our oxygen supply was depleted or suddenly cut off when our umbilical cord was cut, so in that one moment we may not have known if we were about to live or die. (The mechanisms for both life and death are frighteningly similar.) The adaptation to life is driven by catecholamines, which also stimulate the fight or flight mechanism of survival. Thus, in the moment of birth, we may also experience what it is to die. Yet it is not our gift or destiny for the great majority of us to remember this moment.

However, the fear of death or dying never leaves some people and they experience feelings of hopelessness and despair from a very young age. For other people, these feelings can be brought on by later life events, the cumulative effect of which can result in complex mental health issues. Occasionally, in some people, just one single traumatic event can trigger feelings of deep psychological insecurity (Sanders, 2002).

The fear of dying never leaves some people...

But what if at the moment of birth, when the baby is most frightened, some small actions could be taken so as to build that person's resilience for life? These would be small actions that might help build the baby's emotional resilience... resilience that would last a lifetime. These same small actions might also help the new mother build her own resilience so that she would be sustained through her whole experience of motherhood.

The human race has a huge ability to adapt to complex environmental and emotional situations and stimuli. Hence, maternal-infant attachment theories have been hard to prove and are, for some people, difficult to accept because of our multi-faceted approaches to building and sustaining emotional bonds. The subsequent devaluing of the unique moment of birth and those precious unrepeatable early times together has enabled the development of a society which has prioritised medical and institutional needs over the needs of the newborn and his or her mother. Therefore, in our modern, high-tech maternity units, the bond between parents and babies is often made *despite* the care received rather than *because* of it.

In his book *The Scientification of Love* (Free Association Books, 1999) Michel Odent points out the dangers of overlooking these precious moments around birth. He explains how scientific studies have demonstrated a relationship between events during pregnancy and childbirth and babies' later ability to love themselves or others, with devastating consequences for some. He also discusses some research which has tried to explore links between events during childbirth, (such as use of forceps and ventouse, or resuscitation) and the later psychological well-being (or otherwise) of the child as he or she grows up (as measured in terms of autism and suicide). Some researchers, he points out, have felt shunned by the medical community as a result of this research and their shocking findings. Odent postulates that this negative reaction of the medical community may have occurred because establishing detrimental links between birth and later well-being or mental health in adulthood is too emotionally charged politically. Others have also recognised that discussing how the care women receive from some healthcare professionals may contribute to complex relationships is politically sensitive. For example, in her book *Eyes without Sparkle* Hanzak (2005) reflects on her own decline into severe postnatal depression following the birth of her first baby. Her firsthand account clearly illustrates how flippant or insensitive behaviour and comments from healthcare professionals can severely undermine women's confidence and self-esteem during birth and in the early postnatal period.

According to the NICE Antenatal and Postnatal Mental Health Guideline (National Collaborating Centre for Health (NCCH), 2007), approximately 1 in 10 women suffer from postnatal depression. However, the prevalence of depression is no higher in the postnatal period than in the general female population, as women with young children are more prone to depression anyway. However, a recent survey conducted by *Prima Baby* magazine in February 2011 of over 4000 women using the Edinburgh Postnatal Depression Score found that the rate of postnatal depression was double this, with 1 in 5 (20%) of women reporting scores that indicated they were depressed. The boxed vignette below illustrates how the combination of childbirth, complications of childbirth and the attitudes and behaviour of carers can conspire to leave women emotionally vulnerable.

Case study

This is about a woman with no history of mental health problems who went on to develop psychosis after the birth of her three children; it appears in the National Institute for Health and Clinical Excellence (NICE) Guidelines for Antenatal and Postnatal Mental Health (NCCH, 2007, page 66).

Prior to the birth of my children, I had no experience of mental health difficulties. Apart from the great shock and grief I experienced at the sudden death of my mother, when I had to be put under sedation. I positively 'bloomed' throughout my three pregnancies and was totally unprepared for what was to hit me when I experienced psychosis for the first time. My mental distress began in hospital after the birth of my first child. I had an emergency caesarean section following a long labour. An attack of breathlessness within 48 hours of the birth led to me being put on a course of heparin, which soon caused profuse bleeding as the result of a small artery not being tied during surgery. I lost a lot of blood, and my deathly paleness and inability to move very far, or care for my baby without feeling as if I was going to collapse, caused me great anxiety. I was worried that I was going to die and leave my son motherless. No one explained the extent of my anaemia; I was simply told that I'd feel better when I'd had a transfusion, which could not be done until I had come off the heparin. My anxiety increased as the days went by, a situation that was exacerbated by some nurses mocking me because I could not 'cope'. I felt that I was a hopeless mother and I slipped further and further into depression. Not being able to relax or sleep, and feeling continually anxious, the days seemed like weeks.

(This woman goes on to describe her descent into psychosis.)

THE NEED FOR CHANGE IN OUR SYSTEM

In her book *Male and Female* (William Morrow, 1975) Margaret Mead commented that every culture has a subculture around how they treat women during childbirth which reflects the inner values of that particular society's norms. Childbirth in the UK today is as much a rite of passage as in other cultures, although sometimes we just cannot see this because each rite acts as a mirror reflecting back what we are used to seeing. It takes someone with a willingness to look beyond the surface or perhaps not to totally conform with the norms of our society to realise that it can be done differently.

The deeply ingrained, rational scientific culture we live in today suppresses our innate knowledge of how things could improve. We focus on categorising through measuring, counting and documenting what we do, instead of realising deep inside that things must change with regard to our rituals around birth in hospital. It's as if we don't quite know how to engender that change... It's as if we don't know what a new model might look like. Maybe the very reason some people are drawn to midwifery as a profession is because they want that change to occur. Perhaps what drew you was even something to do with what you discovered during your own pregnancy, if you have children of your own. Is it possible that, for some reason, you find it difficult to express the specific improvements you want to see? When our rational, conscious brain engages with the idea that change is needed there is the danger that we will summarily dismiss our ideas as futile.

Challenging cultural norms around childbirth in a society based on a rational, scientific mindset is difficult. The 'evidence-based' mantra of delivery of maternity care implies the assumption that our actions and interventions are immune to cultural influences. It assumes that just because reasons for the care we give women and babies around the moments of birth are reasonable and justifiable, they must be valid. Our very immersion in the currently prevailing mechanistic, dualistic, results-oriented culture has prevented us from naming the problem which exists in maternity care today—and without a name the problem remains elusive. I name the problem to be utilitarian-focused maternity care, where the greater good is seen to take precedence over that of the individual. Utilitarianism in maternity services has led to fragmented and depersonalised care and neglect of the softer emotional, social and community aspects of care, which are so important to the individual woman.

In my view, we need to adopt an holistic approach, embracing spirituality alongside the psychological and physical elements of birth. We need to withdraw from utilitarian maternity care with its Cartesian mind-body split, which has underpinned medical and social aspects of care in recent years. This dualistic approach has allowed maternity-care providers to treat the woman as a baby-making machine, which needs to be assessed, serviced and broken into parts. This approach was supported and extended by Henry Ford's mass early car production model, which enjoyed enormous success in the early 1900s and which had the minimisation of costs as its main goal as well as the 'any colour as long as it's black' production-line model. The transference of both approaches into maternity care was seen in the 1970s when women were considered to be uteri with babies within, which—it was felt—needed to be monitored and checked, measured and delivered on time, just like on a car production line.

> We need to withdraw from utilitarian maternity care
> with its Cartesian mind-body split

Looking back, it's easy to see why a fragmented approach was considered the best way to deliver care in the 1970s and 80s. The sadness for me is that although we've had almost two decades since the government published *Changing Childbirth* (in 1993), which urged continuity, control and choice for women, there has only been sporadic change, with only a few pockets of good practice across the UK. It's very disappointing that in most maternity services, Ford's utilitarian approach is still used, with women being processed through busy labour wards.

It's always difficult to instigate change, so perhaps this explains the slow uptake of the recommendations of the *Changing Childbirth* report from 1993. As Ghandi said, at first people ignore you, then they laugh at you, then they fight you, then you win. I really believe we have to move forward with a different model of care in childbirth in our society. Our current model of maternity care is in danger of being inhumane. The challenge to managers within maternity services is to ensure that women receive high quality, individualised care as part of a consistently delivered service model, even when they give birth in busy maternity units.

> The challenge is to ensure high quality, individualised care

6 welcoming **baby**

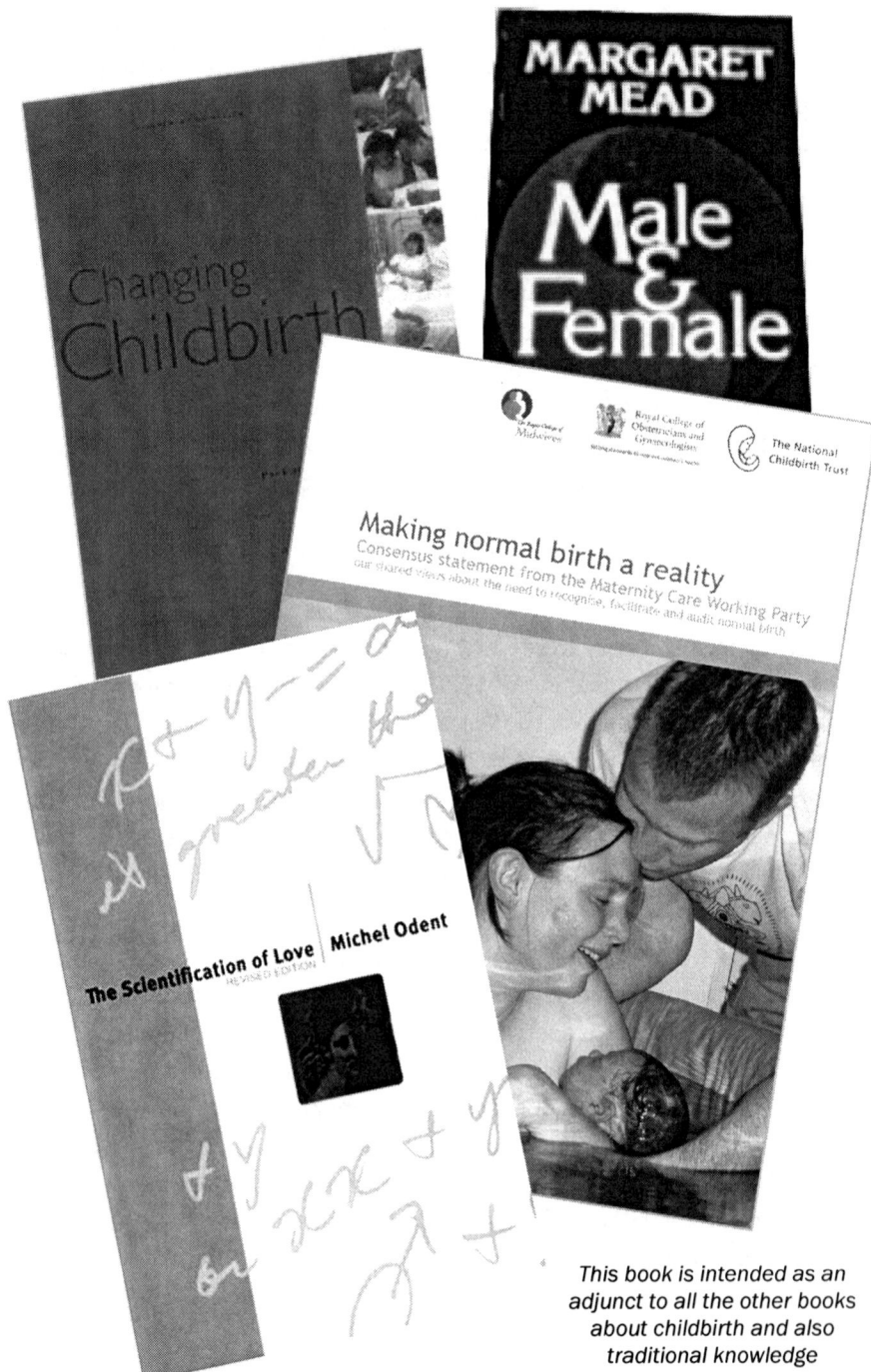

This book is intended as an adjunct to all the other books about childbirth and also traditional knowledge

WHY THIS BOOK?

My purpose is to stimulate debate in order to bring about a profound change in how maternity care is delivered. My deepest interest has always been around midwifery at the moment of birth and in the first few days of a new family. As a community midwife 20 years ago, I was able to support women who I'd got to know during the antenatal period, not only during their births but also in the early postnatal period. This enabled me to find out what was important to women and do my best to deliver it. I have learnt all I know from those women I cared for, while I was trying to translate my reading of academic texts into clinical practice and consider the results—not as a detached observer, as in a research project, but as a fully integrated player in the complex game of life.

In many ways, there's nothing new in what I'm saying, for I'm aware that you may know this information already. Pioneers like Marsden Wagner, who wrote *Pursuing the Birth Machine* (ACE Graphics, 1994), have tried to change our birth culture before me, but we clearly still have a long way to go... The medical profession, in its craving to do the 'right' thing, has concentrated on physical safety. In doing this it may actually have missed the bigger picture and, instead, created unnamed, untamed risks for women, their babies and for society overall. (Incidentally, this book is written from the perspective of childbirth in the UK with occasional references to other areas of practice because it is within the UK that I have developed as a midwife—but similar problems exist around the world, so perhaps this will strike a chord with you, even if you live outside the UK.)

Finally, I should say that this book is intended to be an adjunct to all the other books about childbirth and traditional knowledge that you as a woman, man, mother, father, sister, brother, student midwife, midwife or other health professional have come across. My writing does not aspire to be a replacement for any of your other knowledge of reading... Instead, it aims to become essential reading for anybody who wishes to improve childbirth in our society and appreciate it more. As a book about the importance of childbirth and the baby's first experience of the world, this book focuses on the wonder within us as we journey through life, experiencing the highs and lows of emotions, relationships, successes, failures and even regrets. It also considers the important role that childbirth plays in all of us, both at the beginning of our life's journey and throughout our life. In short, because we still have so far to go in developing a better model of maternity care, this book is a call for change...

The next chapter will continue to explore the situation in obstetrics today.

Exercises

1. Reflect for one minute on the importance of your moment of birth. How is it directly and indirectly linked to your personal identity in terms of your life and also in terms of your place in society? For instance, your date of birth is used as a unique identifier in our culture and most people celebrate their birthday. Horoscopes are also often linked to personality... What's your own perception of the emphasis on time of birth?

2. Try some free writing. In order to facilitate this, have a pen or pencil available, as well as plenty of paper. Also make sure you're somewhere where you won't be disturbed. Then take the following steps:

    - ♥ Close your eyes and think for 10 minutes about what you know about your own birth. (You might want to set a timer so you don't need to check on the time.) To help you start you might like to think about where were you born and how it might have felt to experience your birth as a fetus. What has your mother or family and friends told you about your own birth? Imagine how you were welcomed to the world.

    - ♥ As soon as the 10-minute period is over write for five minutes without lifting the pen from the paper except to start a new page. Don't stop to think and don't worry about using punctuation—just write everything down as it comes into your head, even if it appears to make little sense. Now take a 5-minute break. You will have earned it!

    - ♥ After your break read through what you've written twice. Can you identify any key themes in your writing that may indicate what you value about childbirth practices?

3. Think about how you react to someone who is frightened. What actions do you usually take to try and reassure them? List your three key points from your thoughts.

4. Using the three points above as headings think what you might do differently with a newborn baby if you were to accept that they arrive in the world anxious and frightened.

5. List five words which describe what emotional resilience means to you.

Further reading

Mead M, 1975. *Male and Female*. William Morrow

Murphy J, 2006. *The Power of your Subconscious Mind*. Revised by Dr Ian McMahan. London: Pocket Books.

Odent M, 2005. *The Scientification of Love*. London: Free Association Books.

Wagner M, 1994. *Pursuing the Birth Machine: Search for appropriate birth technology*. London: ACE Graphics.

References

Department of Health, 1993. *Changing Childbirth. Report of the Expert Maternity Group Part 1*. London, HMSO.

Hanzak EA, 2005. *Eyes Without Sparkle: A Journey Through Postnatal Illness*. Oxford: Radcliffe Publishing.

Mead M, 1975. *Male and Female*. William Morrow.

National Collaborating Centre for Health, 2007. *The NICE Guideline on Clinical Management and Service Guidance. Antental and postnatal mental health guideline*. National Collaborating Centre for Health. Website: www.nice.org.uk.

Odent M, 2005. *The Scientification of Love*. London: Free Association Books.

Sanders P, 2002 (3rd ed). *First Steps in Counselling*. Ross-on-Wye: PCCS Books.

Wagner M, 1994. *Pursuing the Birth Machine: Search for appropriate birth technology*. London: ACE Graphics.

2: The situation today

"Every woman needs a midwife, and some need a doctor too."

Sheila Shribman, National Clinical Director for Children, Young People and Maternity Services, DH, 2007

NATIONAL AGENDAS—A SLEEPING BEAUTY

Every single communication counts and good communication is best delivered through relationships. Government policy documents spanning the last 20 years (Midwifery 2020: Delivering Expectations, 2010; Maternity Matters, 2007; Making it Better for Mother and Baby 2007; The National Service Framework (NSF) for Children and Young People, 2004; Changing Childbirth, 1999; and Winterton, 1992) have recommended many changes in the delivery of care to try and improve communication and humanise maternity services. If you look deeper, you will see that the underlying principles which unite all these documents are the delivery of maternity care within and through relationships. I am convinced that if this process is to be successful, then the real art of midwifery needs to meet the science of midwifery in a tangible way, so as to benefit women and their families, midwives and other health professionals. One crucial difference between the NSF and the Changing Childbirth and the Winterton reports is the mandatory nature of policies within the NSF. Back in 2005 I wrote about how the NSF was providing us with an exciting opportunity to take maternity services into the 21st century because of its mandatory nature and because of the far-reaching changes we had seen in other clinical disciplines that had been part of the NSF, such as cancer services (Gould et al, 2005). However, no money came attached to the maternity part of the NSF—unlike cancer services, which had a large boost in funding. Three years after the launch of the NSF, another policy document—Maternity Matters —was released and it reiterated the necessary changes, which had already been outlined. Although the government released some funding for implementing Maternity Matters, access to the money was very difficult for those running maternity services as it was released into the primary care trusts' (PCTs') 'bottom line'—it is the PCTs who commission maternity services—and funds were not necessarily ring-fenced for maternity services (Gould, 2008).

According to the Healthcare Commission 2006, 2007 and 2008 and the Care Quality Commission (CQC) Survey on Maternity Services in 2010, at present these agendas still remain unaddressed, like a sleeping beauty. Many maternity services are still struggling to deliver sensitive maternity services tailored to women's needs. Some services are struggling to change deeply ingrained behaviours and attitudes amongst some healthcare professionals working within our institutions and wider maternity services. There is a discrepancy between theoretically espoused maternity-care values and the reality of the childbirth experience for women and their families. There are also concomitant battles for power and control between the two doctrines of medicalisation and the psycho-social model of care. These battles can result in potentially compromised safety and also affect the psychological and emotional well-being of women and their families, as well as the wider maternity team (King's Fund, 2008). The alleged bullying of healthcare professionals lower down the hierarchy is common within the maternity services, and Kirkham (1999, 2006) has described how midwives often choose conformity with institutional norms even when they know that they are not necessarily doing the right thing. Midwives describe having to go with the flow to avoid bullying behaviour, and they say they feel isolated. It is only when they manage to establish a relationship with some other healthcare professionals that these midwives find the courage to change their own behaviour and speak out when they see other healthcare professionals behaving inappropriately.

In fact, the Nursing and Midwifery Council (NMC) Code (2008) makes it clear that midwives must always put the needs of women and their babies first; that they must act as an advocate for those in their care; that they must not put people at risk; and that they are professionally responsible for their actions and omissions. This means midwives are responsible and accountable for their own behaviour when they choose not to act in the best interests of women and their families and when they choose to ignore their colleagues' behaviour. Yet we know from Kirkham's work that this is exactly what many midwives are doing.

The Healthcare Commission Enquiry in 2006 into the 10 women who died during childbirth at Northwick Park hospital between 2002 and 2005 again highlights these tensions. It also shows that when teamwork between midwives and obstetricians is ineffective, the consequences are tragic—simply because the prevailing culture fosters and tolerates ineffective teamwork.

The professional tensions described in Kirkham's work (1999, 2006) about the culture of maternity services, the reasons why midwives leave the profession described by Ball et al (2002) and the reasons why midwives stay described by Kirkham (2006) are all also referred to in a different way in the King's Fund report into safety in maternity services (2008). This report reinforces the view that good communication and consequent high quality care are best achieved through relationships. It is likely that when a relationship develops between a midwife and a woman, the midwife will find herself more compelled to act as an advocate for the woman... and this will mean that woman-centred care becomes a reality. Thus, the relationship itself puts the woman at the centre of care as described in the NMC Code (2008) and helps midwives to overcome the sometimes immense institutional pressures that they and other healthcare professionals are under to conform to overly medicalised, fragmented, depersonalised care.

This idea is further supported by the Cochrane review (Hatem et al, 2008), which concludes that the delivery of care through established relationships with midwives in a midwifery-led model improves maternal satisfaction and clinical outcomes. Hatem's team reported that there were more normal births, a reduction in interventions and less fetal loss under 24 weeks in a midwifery-led model. Continuity of care and carer themes are interwoven in all the government policies as a vital aspect of high quality, safe maternity care. Nevertheless, continuity of care remains much maligned as unachievable and relatively unimportant amongst many midwives and obstetricians today. However, if these caregivers start getting to know the women they care for, most of them will emotionally engage with the pregnant woman's view of the world. Depersonalisation is rarely sustainable once a relationship has formed. The 'getting through the work' behaviours described by Symonds and Hunt (1994), which can persist today, are then exposed to censure because caring takes priority. If we can stop depersonalisation, many of the current practices in our maternity services—particularly in our labour wards—will become unacceptable and then be forced to change for the better.

A major contributory factor, causing midwives and other healthcare professionals to consciously or subconsciously obstruct change in the delivery of maternity care, is our failure to overcome the fundamental problem that pregnancy and childbirth are seen as an end in themselves in Western society's medical system, and not part of the larger continuum of life and the universe. This leaves people who lead maternity services with a complex conundrum whereby it is not just the process of humanising maternity services that is problematic, but also the process of introducing a clear vision of the wholeness of life. The concept of time, with its 24-hour clock and calendar, is a lens by which we can segment daily life to make it more manageable. Similarly, fragmenting our lives into arbitrary 'time capsules', which we might label 'baby', 'childhood', 'adolescence', 'menarche', 'pregnancy', 'birth', 'motherhood' (or 'parenthood'), 'menopause' and 'pensioner' obscures the fact that people do not experience life in a fragmented way. Life is a complex continuum during which women often find themselves revisiting different issues in different ways over time. And during this ongoing process, relationships are pivotal to well-being and nothing can be broken into isolated segments, simply because everything is interrelated.

Yet the interplay between time and calendar, which allows for scheduling in our daily lives and the time capsules with which we label life, invites the fragmentation of maternity care. This (for the reasons described above) is detrimental to the start of life and reinforces a negative life spiral. We need to move towards trying to support meeting the needs of self-fulfilment and enlightenment throughout the whole of a person's life, from the moment of birth to the moment of death, whatever the circumstances and however the opportunities for this may present themselves. In doing so, we could make a significant positive impact on society's values, behaviours and overall well-being.

The way we treat a woman and her baby during pregnancy and childbirth and the negative correlation this has with the physical, emotional and psychological well-being of the woman, her baby and her wider family, is a massive unrecognised public health issue, even if it is simply a failure to release the potential for empowerment rather than causing harm. To adjust the balance and release the potential for well-being from pregnancy and birth to the wider community we need to reframe how women experience pregnancy and childbirth.

Interestingly, there is a great deal being done to humanise the end of life because of concerns about the cold and inhumane way people have been treated as they necessarily embrace the prospect of death (Department of Health (DH), 2008). In fact, the DH report opens with a quote from Dame Cicely Saunders, Founder of the Modern Hospice Movement: "How people die remains in the memory of those who live on." Although on every level it is vitally important to improve people's experience around birth in a similar way, the wider health gains from humanising the start of life are actually startling in their simplicity, breadth and depth of impact, and it would be easy for these gains to be realised. And while the manner in which we are born lives on in the minds of our mothers, fathers and wider family, it may also be imprinted upon us when we are born.

THE CURSE: INSTITUTIONALISATION

The process of institutionalising all maternity care is a curse. In fact, it is possible to argue that the words which have had the most detrimental impact on maternity services during the last century was the statement contained in the Peel Report (1970) that 100% of women should have their babies in hospital. After all, this statement heralded a massive cultural shift from normality to medicalisation, from community care largely in the home to centralisation of maternity care in hospitals, and it raised obstetrics above midwifery in the professional hierarchy.

Interestingly, this shift towards hospital care was based on assumptions rather than evidence. Many years after the report was written, Marjorie Tew's statistical analysis (in 1998) proved (to her own surprise) that the improved perinatal and maternal outcomes which prompted this recommendation were linked to other medical and social developments such as improved public health, better sanitation and housing, vaccination programmes, the development of antibiotics and the use of blood transfusions. However, so ingrained is hospital birth that even though home birth remains an option for healthy women with healthy pregnancies, the rate remains very low. The Office of National Statistics' latest report (ONS, 2009) states that the homebirth rate fell from 2.9% in 2008 to 2.7% in 2009, with tremendous variations across the country, with 4.1% of women in south-west England giving birth at home compared to 1.3% in the north-east. So the real challenge is that while we still promote choice of place of birth, including home birth, how can we change our focus—and also make our hospitals more fit for purpose?

I am not proposing that we discard our strong rational, scientific basis of working. I am suggesting that our empirical scientific knowledge should be used in tandem with our awareness of the psychosocial changes which are necessary to enhance care... This would mean a very different approach to the one (based *only* on scientific knowledge) which is currently unwittingly undermining quality of care. Following the Peel Report, maternity care has become increasingly institutionalised, despite government policies dating from that time, which have tried to undo the harm that the Peel Report brought to women during pregnancy and childbirth. In fact, recent reconfigurations of maternity services in the United Kingdom are resulting in larger and larger maternity units and this is despite our European counterparts often having better outcomes in smaller maternity units (Bosanquet *et al*, 2005).

Medical routines, rituals and seemingly rational fragmentation of care have become our way of life. Now, as I write, we still have antenatal clinics, labour wards, antenatal and postnatal wards, special care baby units and neonatal intensive care units. Each place has a different focus and once the baby is born the rules change again, with the woman often feeling she has become less important than her baby rather than being seen as an integral person in the mother-baby dyad, within a larger family, as shown by the Care Quality Commission Survey (2010) and the National Childbirth Trust Survey (2010).

In a way, it's as if there are unwritten rules of hospital institutions, which influence this approach. Hotels are often held up as the ideal model for our hospitals to show us how excellent customer care skills can welcome people and make them feel at ease from 'check-in' to 'check-out'—and we are supposed to translate these terms into 'admission' and 'discharge'. Indeed it is true that delivering high quality, personalised care in a rapidly changing population is a challenge facing both hoteliers and maternity care professionals. Reputation is everything in both the hotel industry and the maternity services and we are told that the only real difference should be that maternity services need to emphasise the safety of their care. In fact, based on my experience of staying at a very different type of hotel, which was run as part of a trade union and not as a sole commercial enterprise, I would say that there should be many differences in attitudes and behaviour.

Hoteliers' effective management of discharge procedures in particular is seen as a model for our NHS discharge planning. Hotels, like restaurants, need to be welcoming places so customer care is held in high esteem... After all, the very survival of a hotel depends on recommendations and returning customers. However, the values of an institution are often hidden from those that work within it, only being visible to people who use the service. The hotel I stayed in was very different, though, because it was run by a trade union along socialist collective principles. Its main clientele were trade union workers recuperating after sickness and each guest was paid for by the trade union, which also ran the hotel. The few other paying guests provided additional income, but the hotel was not solely reliant on them for their main business and thus for survival. As the trade union subsidised many of the guests, staff could not see that these people had in fact paid for their stay through years of subscription. In addition, people using the hotel seemed to have lower expectations of customer care because, for them, it appeared to be heavily subsidised. This hotel was located in a quiet seaside resort, overlooking the sea and the bedrooms offered a panoramic view of the sea. Whatever the weather, I would hear the sea outside and realise how powerful nature is. I was so close to the sea that during storms I would sometimes feel frightened of the force that usually slept so near. Yet despite its majestic positioning, the hotel itself lacked lustre. It had a cold, detached feel when you checked in and the staff had an air of being more important than you.

During one memorable evening at this hotel my friends and I were gathering in the nearly empty dining room. The guests recuperating from illness usually ate earlier, then retired to bed. The paying guests preferred to eat later, much to the chagrin of the staff, who wanted to finish early and go home. It would have been the perfect restaurant to dine out with an enemy, as the three courses of the meal were served so quickly we could barely draw breath between mouthfuls of food, let alone strike up witty conversation. If one of us put our fork down, this was a trigger to have our plate removed. Asking for wine was greeted with grunts as it was deemed extra work and a 'delay' in the eating process.

During this particular evening, another friend unexpectedly entered the dining room a little late and came to join us at the table. In the nearly empty dining room she got a chair from another table, brought it over to our table and sat down with us. Suddenly one of the waiters came to our table, looking very disgruntled. Without any attempt to hide his displeasure he told us that we were not to move the chairs ourselves because it could 'do someone out of a job'. It was his job to move the chairs. So not only were we not made very welcome, the unwritten etiquette also had to be followed, or we would risk being told off. The difficulty was that there were no written documents detailing the expectations of behaviour in such an alien environment.

2: The situation today

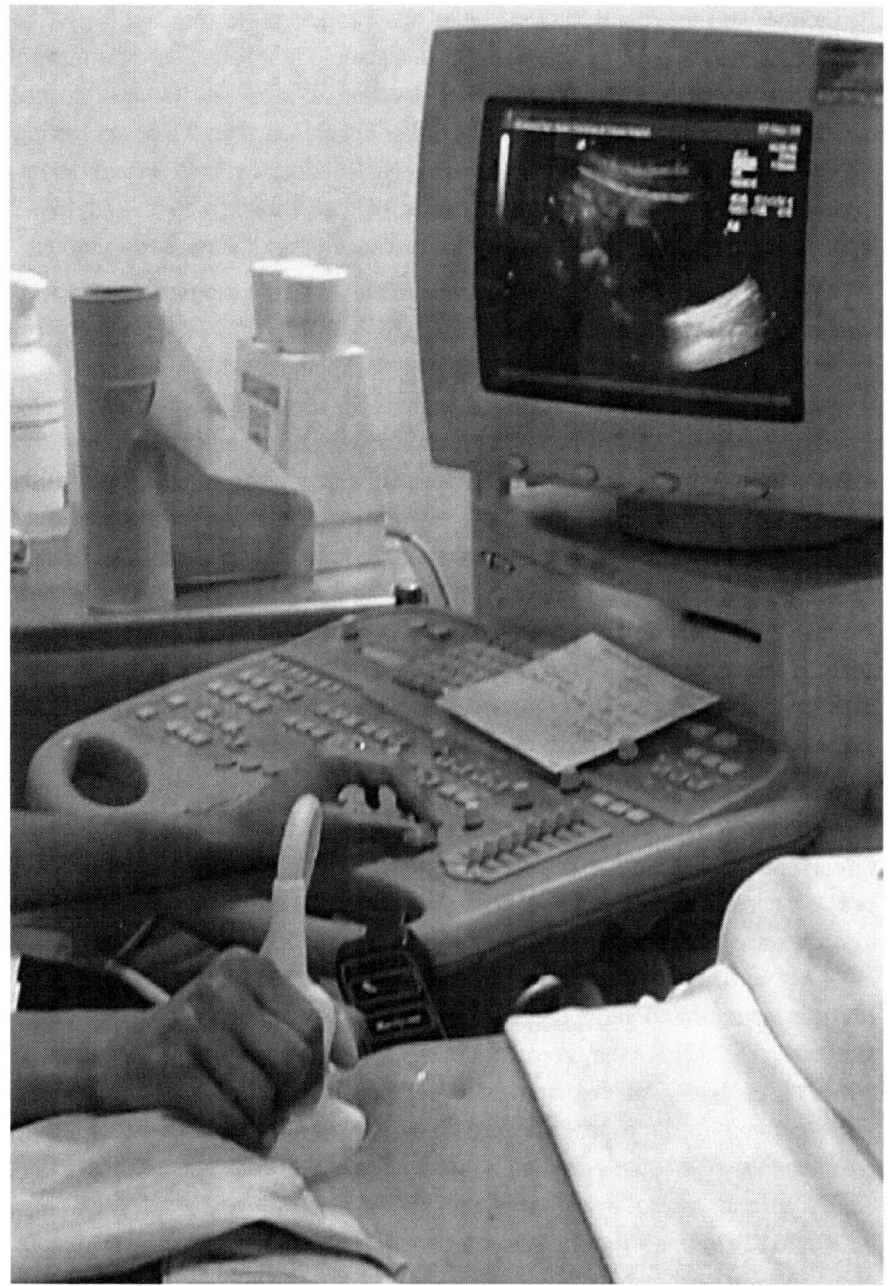

Ultrasound scans are seen by many women as one of the things they are entitled to during pregnancy—but whether or not they are medically needed is rarely considered

By now, you may be wondering what this has got to do with the 'curse' of maternity services, even though some of this institutional behaviour may remind you of our hospitals today. In maternity services, women and families do not overtly pay for health care, so there is a power imbalance, with the power resting with the institution. In his seminal work on organisational dynamics in institutions Goffman (1968) observed that the needs of the 'establishment' and those working within it take precedence over the needs of those it supposedly serves.

Since the early 1990s, there have been efforts to return the power balance to women and their families (DH, 1992, 1993, 2004, 2007.) Offering women choice, continuity and control, as outlined in *Changing Childbirth* (DH, 1993) has become a government mantra that has infiltrated every policy document since then relating to maternity services in England and Wales. Yet even now 'choice' in many cases remains the prerogative of the articulate, educated population and even within this privileged group, it is limited. There are many complex reasons for this, including the fact that women overall want to have their babies fairly close to home, since travelling while in labour is inconvenient and painful at times—plus there is always the risk of the baby being born en route. The emphasis on hospitalised maternity services means resources are concentrated there in the interests of 'safety' and over the past decade many services have suspended their homebirth services, whilst midwives have been redirected to the busy labour wards.

Just as in the case of the socialist trade union hotel I described, maternity care is perceived as 'free' and women and their families are largely happy with it. Offering something 'free' in business has the psychological effect of influencing people's choices and this often distorts their choices in irrational ways as they try to ensure they get the free gift. Women are usually appreciative of their 'free' maternity care, even though it is not free because it is paid for indirectly through National Insurance contributions. Another strange phenomenon occurs with NHS staff precisely because they perceive the maternity services they provide through the NHS as 'free' and this change in perception distorts their attitudes and behaviour—they begin to feel they are doing women a 'favour'. They forget they are members of a team providing a 'service', and that this 'service' should be both safe and nurturing and, where possible, also life-enhancing (Midwifery, 2020, 2010). Women themselves are usually relieved to have survived labour and to have a healthy baby (although this is not the case for a sad minority) so are likely to have lower expectations of care too.

THE AWAKENING: SURVEYS PROMPTING ACTION

In 2007 the Healthcare Commission, now the Care Quality Commission, carried out their first survey on all maternity services in England and Wales (Healthcare Commission 2007, 2008). The results were devastating for many leaders of the maternity services. The survey revealed that institutionalism was rife, with women not being treated with dignity and respect, and that for many the standard of care did not meet national recommendations. It also revealed that there were large disparities across England and Wales. In fact, 20% of all babies born in England and Wales are born in London (LSA, 2010) and sadly London maternity services overall fared the worst of all institutions in these reports. Many aspects of care meant that some midwives' behaviour could have been interpreted as being a breach of the 2008 NMC Code.

This survey carried out by the Healthcare Commission led to numerous working groups and stimulated investment in maternity services. Prior to this the Royal College of Midwives had been campaigning for more midwives for what they believed were chronically underfunded and overstretched maternity services. The survey also catapulted maternity services out of obscurity to the top of the political agenda. Such open scrutiny has since been magnified thanks to increased interest in nursing, midwifery and professional regulation. The role of midwifery supervision has been reconsidered and in April 2009 the Healthcare Commission underwent a metamorphosis into the much more powerful Care Quality Commission, which now regulates health care in England. This intense scrutiny has been painful and is likely to continue to be so, as in maternity services women's experiences are becoming increasingly important, and are being considered alongside the 'safety' of physical and psychological outcomes in pregnancy and childbirth.

The backdrop to the failures of maternity services recorded in the Healthcare Commission's reports (in 2007 and 2008) is that in the NHS in recent years there has been a heavy but rhetorical emphasis on quality of care when quietly, in reality, what has really been important has been financial balance. This has been exacerbated by the clamouring for Foundation Trust status of hospitals in England and Wales. Foundation Trust status puts hospitals more in control of their finances and activities and devolves some regulatory power to the hospital. In order to achieve Foundation Trust status, hospitals needed to achieve financial balance.

The Mid Staffordshire hospital inquiry (Francis, 2010) into failures in a large English hospital illustrated how distorted values can become when whole senior management teams concentrate on financially driven targets and when they value processes above people. Loss of jobs were blamed for the unnecessary deaths of at least 400 people as wards were closed, nursing posts lost and beds squeezed into already overpopulated ward areas. Privacy and dignity were lost. Yet, all the while, care was being delivered by nursing staff who also have an obligation, under their professional code, to ensure that the needs of the people in their care are at the forefront of what they do. There is no clearer indictment than this report. Clearly, simply writing standards for behaviour and care in an official publication by a regulating body does not deliver the advocacy necessary for quality care. In fact, the Mid Staffordshire Report reveals that the whole culture of that Trust had become corrupted and that it was reluctant to accept criticism. A public inquiry has since been set up to establish what exactly happened in the culture within this hospital to ensure that lessons are learnt.

One would think this could not happen within the field of maternity but the Northwick Park Maternity Hospital Report (2006) on the deaths of 10 women who died during childbirth (or within 42 days) states that "despite the good intentions of staff, who were working in very difficult conditions, their practice and ultimately the care that they provided were compromised by the environment and the culture in which they were working. It was an environment that allowed the quality of care to fall below proper professional standards and poor working practices to flourish" (Healthcare Commission, 2006, page 8).

Perverse financial incentives have also been operating in the NHS with births by caesarean sections being generously paid for, while promoting normality has not been similarly rewarded. Even when quality markers are introduced with supposed extra funding, for instance as happened in Commissioning for Quality and Innovation (CQUIN), the 'extra' money is not additional at all. Rather, it is a sum of money withheld until the targets have been delivered. In a wealthy Trust this is barely achievable and in a Trust which is already struggling, withholding funding they might otherwise have is tantamount to forcing them into the very behaviours it is intended they should avoid. Therefore, in the absence of help from financial incentives, what is most important is that women's voices are listened to, from first point of contact to board level and national level.

Promoting normality has not been rewarded within the NHS...

It is likely that, together, these reports and the public inquiry into the Mid Staffordshire NHS Foundation Trust will bring about substantial change in the way hospitals which include maternity services are run and governed in future. If this happens, these hospitals may be able to make progress. To this end, it is essential that any work towards improving maternity services is harnessed positively so as to create a strong, value-driven culture, which puts safety and caring at its heart.

The next chapter will build on the thoughts outlined here and track the development of thinking during the industrialisation of maternity care.

Exercises

1. Take a piece of paper and draw a line down the middle. On one half write 'Medical Model of Care' and on the other half write 'Psycho-social Model of Care'. Now, under each heading, write a list of 10 words which come into your mind when you think of each of the headings.

2. Turn the paper over and make a list of phrases describing how you would like to see your sister, daughter, niece or friend treated during her pregnancy and childbirth.

3. Now look at your lists you have written and write down how you think 'knowing' someone would change the way in which you delivered care. Think of at least three ways in which your approach would change.

4. Reflect on the role 'clock time' plays in compartmentalising our days and, ultimately, our lives.

5. Consider how the concept of 'clock time' exerts control over the delivery of maternity care. How does a focus on 'clock time' affect our attitudes, actions and protocols?

6. Write down what impact, if any, you think the perception of NHS maternity care as 'free' has on the attitudes and behaviours of women and their families using maternity services. Now, write down how you think the perception of NHS maternity care as 'free' affects the attitudes and behaviour of people delivering maternity care.

Further reading

Francis R, 2010. Independent Inquiry into care provided by Mid Staffordshire NHS Foundation Trust.

Tew M, 1998. *Safer Childbirth? A critical history of maternity care.* Free Association Books (3rd revised ed).

Symonds A, Hunt S, 1994. *The Social Meaning of Midwifery.* Palgrave Macmillan.

The King's Fund, 2008. *Safe Birth: Everybody's business.* London: The King's Fund.

References

Ball L, Curtis P, Kirkham M, 2002. 'Why do midwives leave?' Royal College of Midwives.

Bosanquet N, Ferry J, Lees C, Thornton J, Dec 2005. *Maternity Services in the NHS.* Department of Health.

Department of Health, 1993. *Changing Childbirth. Report of the Expert Maternity Group Part 1.* London, HMSO.

Care Quality Commission Survey into Maternity Services, December 2010. Website: www.cqc.org.uk/aboutcqc/howwedoit/involvingpeoplewhouse services/patientsurveys/maternity_services.cfm

Curtis P, Ball L, Kirkham M, 2006. Why do midwives leave? (Not) being the kind of midwife you want to be. *British Journal of Midwifery,* 14(1), 27-31.

Department of Health. House of Commons Health Committee, 1992. *Second Report on the Maternity Services' (The Winterton Report).* London: HMSO.

Department of Health, 2007. *Making it better for mother and baby. Clinical case for change.* London: HMSO.

Department of Health, 2007. *Maternity Matters.* London: HMSO.

Department of Health, 2004. *National Service Framework for Children, Young People and the Maternity Services.* London: Department of Health.

Department of Health, 2008. *End of Life Care Strategy. Promoting high quality care for all adults at the end of life.* London: Department of Health.

Francis R, 2010. 'Independent Inquiry into care provided by Mid Staffordshire NHS Foundation Trust.

Goffman E, 1968. *Asylums.* London: Penguin Books.

Gould D, et al, 2005. Inverting the Hierarchy. *Midwives.* Vol 8, No8, August, pp 362-363.

Gould D, 2008. Money for maternity matters but not as we know it. *British Journal of Midwifery,* Vol 16, No 10, October, p 634.

Hatem M, Sandall J, Devane D, Soltani H, Gates S, 2008. Midwife-led versus other models of care for childbearing women. *Cochrane Database Systematic Review.* Oct 8;(4):CD004667.

Healthcare Commission, 2006. *Investigation into 10 maternal deaths at, or following delivery at, Northwick Park Hospital, North West London.*' London: Commission for Healthcare Audit and Inspection.

Healthcare Commission, 2007. *Women's experiences of maternity care in the NHS in England. Key findings from a survey of NHS trusts carried out in 2007.* London: Commission for Healthcare Audit and Inspection.

Healthcare Commission, 2008. *Towards better births: a review of maternity services in England. The key findings and recommendations from our comprehensive review of maternity services in England Commission for Healthcare Audit and Inspection.*

Kirkham M, 1999. The culture of midwifery in the NHS in England. *Journal of Advanced Nursing* 30(3): 732-9.

Kirkham M, 2006. *Why do midwives stay?* University of Sheffield.

Midwifery 2020 UK Programme (2010) Midwifery 2020: Delivering Expectations. Edinburgh: Midwifery 2020 UK Programme. Website: http://midwifery2020.org.uk/documents/M2020Deliveringexpectations-FullReport2.pdf

Nursing & Midwifery Council, 2008. The Code, Standards of conduct, performance and ethics for nurses and midwives. London: Nursing & Midwifery Council. Website: www.nmc.org.uk

Office of National Statistics (ONS), 2009. *Live births in England and Wales by characteristics of birth.*

Peel Report, 1970. Standing Maternity and Midwifery Advisory Committee. 'Domiciliary midwifery and maternity bed needs: report of a sub-committee.' London: HMSO.

Symonds A, Hunt S, 1994. *The Social Meaning of Midwifery.* Palgrave Macmillan.

The King's Fund, 2008. *Safe Birth: Everybody's business.* London: The King's Fund.

Tew M, 1998. *Safer childbirth? A critical history of maternity care.* Free Association Books (3rd revised ed).

3: A developing outlook towards maternity care

"... we have no more reason to think it is our mind which causes movements which we do not experience as being guided by our will, than we have to judge that there is a soul in a clock, which makes it display the time."

René Descartes (1596-1650), French philosopher and writer

THE IDEA OF THE 'MIND-BODY' SPLIT

If we are to truly welcome babies into the world a major cultural shift is required in terms of the way in which midwifery and maternity services are perceived and delivered—from both a psychological and a physical perspective. Truly welcoming babies requires a withdrawal from the Cartesian mind-body split that continues to fuel medical and social aspects of health care.

Dualism, an understanding that the mind and spiritual aspects are somehow separate from the body, has been around since the early Greek philosophers Aristotle and Plato. This concept was embedded further into Western psyche by the philosopher René Descartes, who famously said: "I think therefore I exist" in his *Discourse on Method and the Meditations* (Penguin Classics, reprinted 1998). As a result of his analysis of the way the mind can reflect and think about activities going on in and around the body, he came to the conclusion that there must therefore be a split between mind and body. This was later to have far-reaching consequences in the future development of health care for emerging rational scientific medicine and it was to have an important influence on childbirth practices. In fact, around the time of Descartes there was a phenomenal rise in rational scientific thought which now underpins today's rational scientific model. Descartes' views led to the body being treated as a machine, the sum of which can easily be broken down into parts. And as we learnt more about anatomy, physiology and physics, our understanding of what makes the body work became increasingly complex and also fragmented.

The notion of a divided mind-body interface, which was first expressed in 1637, persisted up until the 1980s. Then the publication of Candace Pert's seminal work *Molecules of Emotion, Why You Feel the Way You Feel* (Simon and Schuster, 1997) proved to our rational scientific predecessors that emotions do in fact exert an influence on the physiology of organs and cells and that the way our body responds has a profound effect on our mind. Pert's laboratory work created the biomolecular basis which led to her theory of 'bodymind'. Interestingly, by combining mind and body, she describes how we as humans function as a unified psychosomatic network, giving and transmitting information at a molecular level and thereby controlling our health and physiology. Pert was one of the pioneers of a new medical discipline known as 'psychoneuroimmunology'. Pert's theories about the unconscious mind and its influence on psychosomatic illness, happiness, and wellness, led to her being awarded the Theophrastus Paracelsus Prize for Holistic Medicine in Switzerland in 2008. Nevertheless, this is still relatively new territory in research terms because it usually takes 10 to 15 years for research evidence to translate into practice. To slow this process down further, the field of psychoimmunology is still very new so the full impact of this ground-breaking knowledge is still to be felt at the clinical care level.

AN INADEQUATE APPROACH TO ANALYSIS

We can see that if a machine approach is applied to the body, different body parts lend themselves to being reviewed separately and so are serviced and possibly fixed in isolation to the greater whole. In early midwifery and obstetrics textbooks, the oversimplification and fragmentation of the complex interplay between emotional, hormonal and physiological processes of birth are graphically depicted in the teaching of 'The Three Ps'. Within the pages of these texts, which date from the 1980s and possibly before, and which even persist to this day, there are descriptions of labour which refer to the role of 'The Three Ps'. These 'Three Ps' refer to 'powers' (uterine contractions), 'passage' (pelvis or birth canal) and 'passenger' (the fetus). Note, though, that in this model the woman herself is not mentioned at all. Where is she in the process of childbirth? In what might be seen as a development—if it were not for the fact that the model is over-simplistic and flawed—a fourth 'P' was later added, representing the 'psyche'. Presumably this was a recognition that the woman herself does indeed have a role in childbirth as a whole person.

THE FORGOTTEN POWER OF THE PLACEBO

By removing the uncertainties and variations that individuals might exert through their mind, it was possible to carry out scientific experiments so as to identify the' truth' of the mind-body relationship... or split. After all, the rational scientific model is really the simplification of life circumstances so that the best clinical experiments can be conducted. Testing one thing at a time in a set way, scientific researchers have been trying to reproduce laboratory conditions in the real world. In this respect, the National Institute for Health and Clinical Excellence (NICE) sees the randomised controlled trial (RCT) as the gold standard for evidence-based medicine in general and for nursing and midwifery practice in particular—and the medical profession at large takes the same view. RCTs usually involve one treatment or intervention, groups which are as alike as possible and the measurement of predetermined outcomes (i.e. studies are carried out *prospectively*). Usually there is a control group which does not receive the intervention so as to prevent the well-documented placebo effect from blurring the findings.

A placebo is a substance containing no medication which is given to reinforce a personal expectation. Interestingly, the RCT works hard to eliminate the placebo effect and yet the placebo effect itself may have great beneficial effects, especially in pregnancy and childbirth. A great example of a placebo is from the Walt Disney film *Dumbo*. The baby elephant with big ears, who is called Dumbo, is able to fly as long as he holds his 'magic' feather, which was given to him by another character, Timothy the Mouse. When Dumbo drops the feather, he no longer believes he can fly and as he is falling Timothy confesses that the feather was not magic at all. He reveals that he had tricked Dumbo into believing he could fly—which meant that he was actually able to! Take away the belief that something is possible and unhindered doubt and lack of confidence will stop people from doing things they might otherwise be capable of. Arguably, while our oversimplification of medicine is one of our biggest achievements, it is also one of the greatest failures of the modern healthcare system. While it has caused great gains in technical knowledge, expertise and the development of technology, it has also belittled women's inner knowledge and confidence. Rebuilding this is going to take more than a feather... It will take visionaries who believe we have to do things differently.

Rebuilding women's confidence is going to take vision

CARTESIAN ASSESSMENT OF THE BABY AT BIRTH

Another example of the reductionist scientific approach to childbirth can be seen in the widely accepted protocol which involves recording Apgar scores at birth as a measurement of the well-being of the baby soon after birth. The Apgar score was devised by Virginia Apgar in 1952 and was first published in 1953. It came about when Apgar, an anaesthetist in the USA, felt there was an emphasis on assessing the mother's well-being but not necessarily that of the baby. The Apgar score epitomises the alienation that a concentration on narrowed medicalised measurements of care can represent. It also shows how once rational scientific 'scoring' is begun and embedded into care patterns (even if it is of little real use) it continues to be incorporated into care later on.

Once scoring is embedded into care, it continues to be incorporated

The Apgar score is inadequate because it assesses only five aspects of the newborn's complex adaptation to life outside the womb: breathing, heart rate, response to stimuli, skin colour and muscle tone. Each attribute is given the same importance and marked out of two, with each possible score being 0, 1 or 2, meaning that the highest possible Apgar score is 10. As can be seen from Virginia Apgar's original paper on this approach to assessment, there are considerable questions around the relevance of each of the categories chosen, especially the response to stimuli. We no longer recommend routine oral or nasal suctioning, although the response to stimuli scoring was mainly based on this practice, and we no longer see the spontaneous passing of urine or meconium as being positive—although Apgar did in fact record this as being another positive response to stimuli. Apgar also acknowledged that the assessment of a baby's colour was one of the weakest elements of the scoring system but of course it is still weighted equally alongside the other four signs. When reviewed critically, then, it is difficult to imagine that the Apgar score might be used as anything more than a retrospective measure of well-being and even if it is used in that way it must be viewed as a pseudo outcome measure.

Even Apgar herself acknowledged in her original paper that she wanted the 'reestablishment of simple, clear classification or 'grading' of newborn infants which can be used as a basis for discussion and comparison of the results of obstetric practices, types of maternal pain relief and the effects of resuscitation.' She also acknowledged that the idea of a 'scoring system' came out of her work with drug addicts. Scores of 8, 9 or 10 equated to the baby being in a good condition, while those of 0,1 or 2 indicated a poor condition and babies who scored somewhere in between were assessed as being in a fair to moderate condition.

As you probably also know, the Apgar scoring assessment is traditionally undertaken at 1 minute, 5 minutes and 10 minutes. It should not be scored before 1 minute as many babies are still adapting to life and a disproportionately large number of healthy babies would be given a low Apgar score if the assessment were undertaken too early. However, in practice, there are some babies who need immediate active resuscitation rather than waiting for the full minute to make the Apgar assessment. These are the babies who look white or pale, make no effort to breathe, are very floppy on handling, often with fixed staring eyes and who, on assessment, have no heart rate. These babies need immediate intervention to resuscitate them and waiting one minute may well be harmful. Furthermore, during resuscitation of the newborn, regular assessment should take place approximately every 30 to 60 seconds considering breathing (including the presence of chest movement in response to lung ventilation), skin or mucus membrane colour, and heart rate. Response to stimuli and muscle tone, although relevant to the whole picture, are not the cardinal signs which drive resuscitation efforts today. Yet the Apgar score does not weigh its answers according to relevance to need for resuscitation or overall well-being. It also gives no credence to a baby being alert, looking around and seeking eye contact.

Still, the Apgar score is so engrained into maternity care that all babies born in the UK with a healthcare practitioner present now have an Apgar score allocated to them at 1 and 5 minutes, with most also having a 10-minute score recorded. As I've explained, the Apgar score's absolute relevance in clinical practice is questionable, even within the rational scientific model, and it does not take into account the many other factors which play out at the time of birth for the baby. For instance, although the Apgar score is scored out of 10 even for the first-minute assessment, in reality most healthy babies only score 9 as they still have blue peripheries, i.e. their hands and feet. As a result, a newborn can virtually never score 10 at one minute, even though he or she may be extremely healthy.

Apgar score table modified from Virginia Apgar (1953)

SIGN AND SCORE	0	1	2
Heart rate	Absent	Less than 100	Over 100
Respiratory effort	None	Weak, irregular or 'grunting'	Good respiratory effort; crying
Colour	Pale; white	Blue	Pink
Muscle tone	Limp	Moderate; still	Good; moving
Response to stimuli	None	Reduced; poor	Brisk

In fact, the Apgar score has been adopted worldwide as a measure of the baby's well-being at birth and it remains a major assessment tool today. Although the intention was to facilitate a systematic review of the baby's condition at birth rather than act as a comparative tool, it has become used as a comparative tool in many studies. These studies range from trying to identify which babies will go on to have cerebral palsy to measuring the difference in the babies' well-being between those whose mothers smoked and those whose mothers did not—so it has clearly become a pseudo-outcome measure. However, there are criticisms that the Apgar score lacks specificity, since some newborn infants may have a low Apgar score but still be healthy. Furthermore, the Apgar score is also poorly correlated to long-term outcomes, and perhaps a greater emphasis should be put on cord blood gas analysis to indicate babies who have had intrapartum asphyxia than on the Apgar score. In reality, the Apgar score is most often done retrospectively, not contemporaneously. For whilst clinicians look for the signs of well-being, i.e. breathing or respiratory effort, colour, good heart rate, movement and muscle tone, they do not necessarily score them at the same time.

One study conducted by Clark and Hakanson (1988) showed that there are large differences in the way in which different types of professional groups assess Apgar scores. Neonatologists and paediatricians achieved most consistency when given case studies to review, whilst obstetricians and 'obstetric nurses' (the study was undertaken in America where there are very few midwives) had the lowest consistency ratings. Originally the person facilitating the birth was not supposed to be the person assessing the baby's condition as it was felt that there may be an element of bias, particularly if there was a poor outcome, when the person assessing was also the person caring for the woman in labour. This emphasis on an independent objective view of the baby's Apgar assessment has been lost in modern maternity care. In another study carried out in 2006 (O'Donnell, *et al*) researchers again found great discrepancies between different clinicians, known as interobserver discrepancies, in all four signs of the Apgar score on the same babies. In this study, clinicians were played videotapes of babies at birth and asked to assess the Apgar score. Differences in assessment persisted regardless of the condition of the babies—even though previously it had been asserted that Apgar scoring was more accurate with well babies. Despite this growing evidence that the Apgar score is an inadequate measure of well-being, it continues to be used in maternity units and, more worryingly, as an outcome measure of benefits in research studies.

In the case of Apgar scoring, as elsewhere in maternity care, the mother-baby link is devalued and fragmented into something which we claim we can measure, even though measuring of the Apgar score is futile since it is so inaccurate. Time spent on teaching, learning and assessing Apgar scores not only detracts from time spent trying to build sensitive, emotionally receptive and responsive maternity services... it also reinforces a fragmented model of care which values numbers and processes above real people and relationships. Interestingly, though, in the UK it is most likely the midwife who often decides and records the Apgar score—even though she (or he) is most likely to be the champion of change in this respect.

Nevertheless, despite some lone voices recognising the limitations of this fragmented approach, there has as yet been no real challenge to this simplistic view of assessing the baby's well-being. There has been no real challenge to this system which is clearly focused on physical adaptation and which ignores the emotional and relationship elements of successful adaptation to life.

In fact, as long ago as 1993 obstetrician Michelle Harrison suggested that midwives might better be able to understand the baby's short- and long-term well-being if they took a broader look at those first few precious minutes and hours following birth, and at the relationships and emotions in the birth room. She suggested asking the following questions to make a broader assessment of the adaptation to life facing the baby and his or her mother, and other significant people, including fathers:

- ♥ Do those in the room feel close to each other and the baby?
- ♥ Does the baby look healthy?
- ♥ Does the baby feel welcomed into the world?
- ♥ Does the baby make eye contact?
- ♥ Is the baby curious?
- ♥ Does the baby respond to touch, to voice, to being held?
- ♥ What is the mother's mood? Happy? Depressed? Frightened?
- ♥ What is the baby's mood? Happy? Depressed? Frightened?
- ♥ Was the baby smiling in the birth canal?
- ♥ Does this mother feel good about herself after this birth?
- ♥ Is the mother ready to move on to the next phase of their relationship, whether that is together or apart?
- ♥ Was love present?

These key questions could be transposed into birth dimensions to help build the baby's relationship with his or her mother and other significant people. Usually a woman will choose very significant people in her life to be her birth partner(s) or to visit soon after the baby's birth. Her choice of birth partner(s) will in fact often, but not always, give us a glimpse into who can most positively influence how well this woman and her baby will grow together.

In exploring these dimensions, we can start to move beyond a production line approach to birth and embrace the emotional and relationship elements of care which are crucial to high quality maternity care. Further questions are provided in the table below so as to facilitate further evaluation of the mother-baby dyad. Note that the birth impact dimensions are written assuming that the woman is physically well. However, they can also be of use to women who are unwell immediately following birth as they give a platform for midwives and family members to facilitate a stronger relationship between mother and baby once the woman is well enough. These birth impact baby dimensions (used alongside Harrison's questions) could also be used to engender a stronger father-baby relationship, particularly if some or all of the suggestions for action are taken on board.

32 welcoming baby

Birth impact on baby dimensions modified from Harrison 1993	Harrison's questions	Actions of the midwife or other birth attendant(s)
Health	Does the baby look healthy? Does the baby make eye contact? Is the baby curious?	A baby exhibiting all these characteristics will be healthy and focus should be on facilitating an early, quality relationship with the baby's mother (and father). Encourage skin-to-skin contact between mother and baby. Take a step back so you can provide some space, privacy, warmth and quiet. Give gentle encouragement to the mother, if necessary, highlighting to her various cues which show how the baby is curious about her new parents (e.g. eye contact).
Love and attachment	Do those in the room seem to feel close to each other and also to the baby? Does the baby seem to feel welcomed into the world? Did love appear to be present? Does the baby respond to touch, to his or her mother's (or father's) voice, and to being held?	Reflect on how the environment and events during labour may have impacted on the amount of love in the birthing room. If there is no feeling of love in the room, try describing to the new mother the baby's response to touch, her voice and to being held. If this is done in a positive way, this could lighten the mood and create a feeling of love. Ensure appropriate privacy and overtly show loving gestures to the mother and her new baby. Emotions are contagious so be ready to emotionally lift a negative atmosphere. Remember that the use of body language may be more powerful than words, which may sound contrived or awkward.

A table linking answers to various key questions to appropriate action (Part 1—see part 2 on the facing page)—based on Harrison, 1993

3: A developing outlook towards maternity care 33

Birth impact on baby dimensions modified from Harrison 1993	Harrison's questions	Actions of the midwife or other birth attendant(s)
Mothering, self-esteem and confidence	Does this mother feel good about herself after this birth? Is the mother ready to move on to the next phase of her relationship, whether that is together with her baby or separately (in the case of an adoption) What is the mother's mood? Does she seem elated? Happy? Relieved? Depressed? Frightened?	Notice how the woman behaves, expresses herself and describes herself soon after the birth. Be ready to quickly intervene with positive reassurance to mitigate against any negative thoughts being embedded into her psyche regarding her actions or behaviour during labour. Be aware of the power of flippant comments at this emotionally raw stage of transition to motherhood, for women most often remember everything happening around the time of birth for the rest of their lives. This can also have a powerful impact on their confidence and self-esteem. Ensure your actions are aimed at building the woman's self-esteem and confidence, even more so if the mother is not feeling elated or good about herself. Encourage other birth partners and attendants to do the same.
Baby's mood	What is the baby's mood? Does he or she appear to be happy? Content? Depressed? Frightened?	Utilise skin-to-skin contact even if the baby seems unhappy. It is the surest way to soothe an unhappy or frightened baby. If the mother is unable or unwilling to hold her baby, see if you can encourage someone else to do this until the baby is calmer or the mother well enough. Then encourage the mother to do hold her new baby. Encourage frequent skin-to-skin contact with the mother, especially if the baby or the mother's mood were not optimal around the moment of birth.

A table linking answers to various key questions to appropriate action (Part 2)—based on Harrison, 1993

THE INDUSTRIALISATION OF MATERNITY CARE

Within the strong, simplistic and mechanistic scientific model of maternity care, pregnancy and childbirth care have also been associated with a valuation of industrialisation, as already noted. During the industrialised production of goods, with newly developed automated production lines, the product is passed on a conveyor belt through a myriad of workers, each of whom undertakes a particular aspect of production over and over again. The interest in Henry Ford's car production line remains today and is now honoured with the term 'Fordism'. Ford's exploitation of technology such as the conveyor belt and his idea to use people to do the same task over and over again was ostensibly introduced to reduce the inefficiencies of highly skilled craftsmen who did mundane work (as well as skilled work) which other workers could do for them. Ford's system meant that it was possible to produce cars more efficiently at much lower cost. This revolutionised the public's perception of the car and as cars became more affordable, they also became increasingly popular.

However, Ford's approach sacrificed some elements of quality in order to enhance consistency and maximise output for the lowest cost Model T. Ford famously said: "You can have any colour as long as it's black." Choice was not a priority...

Full industrialisation and medicalisation of maternity care started with the Peel Report in 1970. Until this point, the majority of maternity care had been delivered by midwives in the community with home birth being seen as normal. However, the Peel Report recommended that all women should give birth in hospitals and, accepting this recommendation, maternity hospitals increased the number of beds they had available. This opened the doors for medicalised care at the expense of the social model of midwifery. The hospital and its staff, rather than the woman in her home, became the central focus.

The move from home to hospital enabled the medical profession, which dominated the hospitals at that time and which remains very powerful even today, to virtually take full control of maternity care and midwifery in a way that even the Midwives Act (1902) had not quite enabled them to do. The Midwives Act was in fact a life and death act for midwifery in that it created the role of the midwife in statute but at the same time embalmed midwifery in a subservient role at the service of the medical profession, stipulating that midwives were under the supervision of doctors.

In order to cope with the sudden increased demand for hospital beds, given the shift from home-based care to hospitalisation, the industrial model crept unhindered into maternity care. Instead of seeing the whole woman's journey through pregnancy and childbirth, healthcare providers 'specialised' in different areas. In hospitals, the clinic and ward model of the sick had to be used, instead of a majority of well women experiencing a peak life event. The transition was not smooth so to make this new style of care acceptable to women, the riskier side of pregnancy and birth was emphasised. Later, some said that this emphasis on risk had been overdone. Overall, translated into maternity care, Fordism meant that antenatal care was now delivered in hospitals and that intraparum practices were based on the needs of doctors and not on those of women.

In the early 1980s when I first started practising midwifery, women would wait in large antenatal clinics to be seen by a doctor. When they arrived they would be required to remove all of their clothes, including their underwear, to put on a hospital gown, so that they would be 'ready' for the doctor's examination, which often included a vaginal examination. Comparing this with today's practices, it seems astounding and it is a prime example of non-evidence-based production line care where respect for the woman as a person was sidelined for the sake of efficient use of the doctor's time. This maximisation of time efficiency arguably also led to the centralisation of women in labour on labour wards so that there could always be access to doctors 'just in case'. Midwives and all women with one particular condition—in this case those in labour—were confined to one area and women who'd had their baby were transferred to the postnatal ward. Very soon a maternity production line was up and running. Efficiency was further enhanced by the specialisation of midwives, some of whom preferred antenatal care, some labour and some postnatal care, and compounded the fragmentation of care. Because of increased perceived risks of pregnancy and childbirth and the use of technology, labour wards came to be seen as central to this hierarchy of services and 'admission rooms' were used so that women could have a full assessment before being directed to the appropriate area. Increasingly, centralisation and fragmentation of care became the model across the UK.

However the move to hospital for maternity care did not have to happen in this manner and fragmentation did not necessarily have to follow. If doctors had had a holistic approach they could have built hospitals to accommodate women at whatever stage of their pregnancy, much like free-standing birth centres often do today.

THE DEVELOPMENT OF A NEW PERSPECTIVE

As early as the mid 1950s there was growing discontent with maternity care. In 1956 the Natural Childbirth Association was established and its original aims still echo much of what is required from maternity care today. In 1961 it became a registered charity called the National Childbirth Trust (NCT). However, it was not until the early 1990s that this pressure group began to influence change in maternity care by using its extensive evidence built up over time through research into women's experiences. (See the table below, outlining the original aims of the NCT.)

The original aims of the NCT

- That women should be humanely treated during pregnancy and in labour, never hurried, bullied or ridiculed.
- That husbands should be present during labour if mutually desired.
- That analgesia should not be forced on women in childbirth (and) nor should labour be induced merely to save time.
- That more emphasis should be given to self-regulated breastfeeding and rooming-in allowed if the mother wants it, and that future maternity units should be designed with this in mind.
- That a mother trained for natural childbirth should be allowed and encouraged to carry out her training fully during labour.
- That all mothers should be encouraged to use natural childbirth for the benefit of themselves and their babies and that posters to this effect should be displayed at all antenatal clinics.
- That the idea fostered by many medical people today that natural childbirth includes routine internal examination; routine administration of analgesia, routine episiotomy should be dispelled.
- As childbirth is not a disease it should take place in the home wherever possible. If impossible the maternity units should be homely and unfrightening and in no way connected with hospital.

From the National Childbirth Trust website: www.nct.org.uk/about-nct/our-history [accessed 30 August 2011]

Nevertheless, the combination of the success of the production line in industrialisation and the rational scientific approach in medicine led to depersonalisation in maternity care. Increasingly, throughout the 1970s and 80s, women were broken down into uteri which had fetuses within, that needed to be monitored, checked, measured and delivered on time, moving through maternity services with 'experts' waiting in line to service them.

In the hospital environment, the rational scientific model was incredibly powerful. Midwives voices became weak as doctors started to undertake almost all midwifery care apart from postnatal care which has never, even today, attracted a great deal of medical attention. Michel Odent also (2002) argues that advances in the development of plastics, anaesthesia and surgical training for obstetricians in the 1960s and 70s further transformed birth into a surgical event as the caesarean section became safer. On account of this, fetal monitoring was emphasised because the technology had been developed to allow continuous electronic fetal monitoring to take place. The effects of these seemingly unrelated events were profound and remain palpable in maternity services today.

Ann Oakley, a prominent feminist and sociologist, joined the movement to challenge the depersonalisation and overmedicalisation of maternity care from the 1980s onwards. She described the current maternity services in unforgiving detail and analysed the power and control that had become embedded within them. She used her feminist research and writings to tell the story of how the essence and power of womanhood had been eroded through the control of childbirth at the hands of a largely male-dominated medical profession. Some of her books were scathingly titled to help publicly emphasise the power play and political nuances of maternity care provision at that time. These included *Women Confined: Toward a Sociology of Childbirth* (1980). Of course, 'confinement' is an-old fashioned term for labour and birth which is linked to a time when women were expected to spend long periods of time in bed. It is a medical term that was still in frequent use in the 1980s. In fact, 'home confinement' is a term still used today, despite numerous attempts to remove such antiquated language from the midwifery and medical profession and instead use the term 'home birth'. *Women Confined* was followed by the *The Captured Womb: A history of the medical care of pregnant women* and, together, these books summoned up the overwhelming sense of powerlessness and anger that women receiving care during pregnancy and childbirth were beginning to complain about. Ann Oakley gave women and midwives a much-needed voice and encouragement to change during the 1980s and beyond.

However it was to be another decade before the earliest signs of political change were to appear in the area of maternity care.

> It was not until 1991 that women had a voice in maternity care

In fact, it was not until 1991 that women had a voice in maternity care. At last they started to be heard, rebelling against the Fordism reductionist model of maternity care. The National Childbirth Trust, which had now been increasing its influence as a user lobbying group, was invited by Nicholas Winterton (who was then leading a governmental review of maternity services) to comment on maternity services so its extensive research could be used to good effect. Nicholas Winterton also chose to elicit women's views so he visited maternity units. His report recommended far-reaching changes and included a recommendation for a social model of maternity care. It was the first Department of Health document to refer to pregnancy and childbirth as a 'manifestation of health' (Winterton Report,1992) and as a healthy social event for the majority of women, and not as an illness. This was in complete contrast to the risk-generated view of obstetrics which holds that pregnancy and birth are only normal in retrospect. In its response to the Winterton Report, the Government commissioned another review which was published in 1993, called *Changing Childbirth*.

Changing Childbirth (1993) talked about the three 'Cs' (rather than the three 'Ps'), namely 'choice', 'control' and 'continuity' of care and carer. It also discussed flexible, woman-centered, evidence-based care wtihin a social model. This view has largely driven public policy on maternity services since that time, as seen in the Department of Health publications of *The National Service Framework for Children, Young People and Maternity Services* (2004) and *Maternity Matters* (2007). However, even if we can clearly see how industrial and medical advances may have led to fragmented care in the 1970s and 80s, it is difficult to see why it was considered the best way to deliver care. In the majority of maternity services around the country (and indeed around the world), the Fordism approach remains valued as women are processed through busy labour wards. In most places individualised care is only given incidentally, more as a token acknowledgement than as a central part of care.

> It is difficult to see why fragmented care was considered the best way to deliver care in the 1970s and 80s

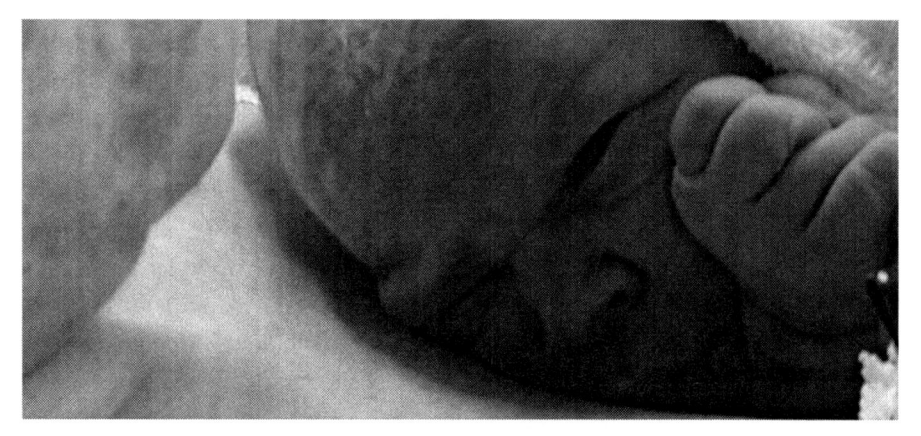

3: A developing outlook towards maternity care 39

The 'passenger' arrives (see page 25)

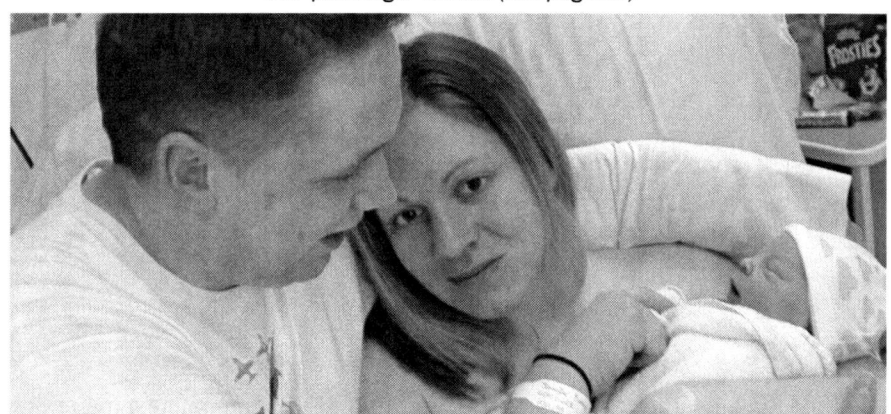

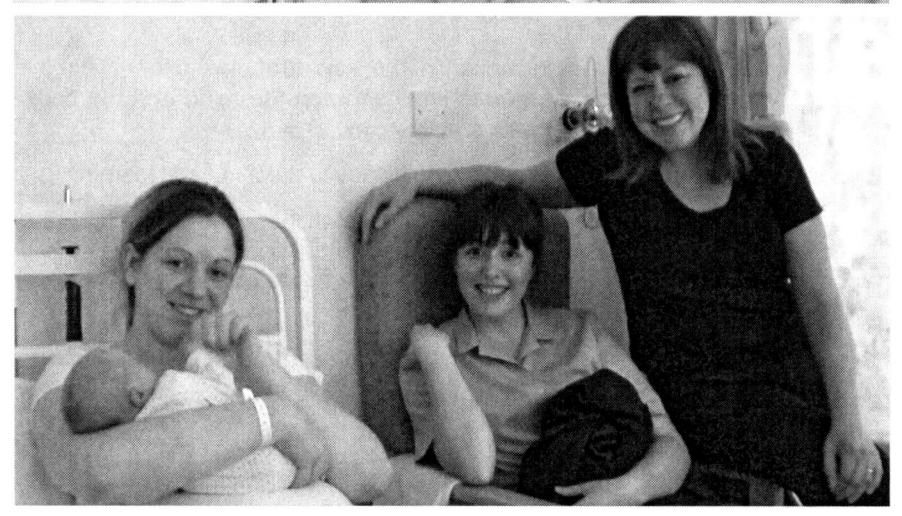

The 'passenger' is held... or is this a passenger after all?... or something else entirely?

The underlying influence of industrial production lines still permeates the delivery of maternity care, sometimes subtly and sometimes more overtly. Even the increasing centralisation of guidelines based on evidence-based care (through NICE) has been disappointing, since this body continues to give more credence to reductionist randomised controlled trials than to other qualitative measures. Maternity service reconfigurations continue to involve centralisation in larger and larger maternity units, with larger and more technical labour wards. Pregnancy itself has become a moving conveyer belt of medical testing and intervention from the time when the woman first finds out she is pregnant until after the birth of her baby, whereupon she is deposited back into the social world of motherhood... but at what cost to women and society?

> The underlying influence of industrial production lines still permeates the delivery of maternity care, sometimes subtly and sometimes more overtly

In the next chapter I shall further expand on developments within the car manufacturing industry and consider how they continue to have far-reaching effects on the delivery of care in maternity services.

Exercises

1. Take three minutes to focus on the key attributes underpinning a maternity service based on 'Cartesian dualism'.
2. Now take three minutes to focus on the key attributes underpinning a maternity service which recognises links between the mind and the body, i.e. which is based on a 'bodymind' philosophy.
3. List three examples of reductionist approaches to teaching and learning.
4. Using the three examples of reductionist approaches to teaching and rate each of them out of 5 (1 is high and 5 is low) with regards to how well these each reflect the lived experience of childbirth.
5. Think of an example from your own life when the 'placebo' effect has been used to boost your own confidence.
6. With a partner or on your own using the title 'The use of placebo is unethical in maternity care' debate the advantages and disadvantages of placebos.

Further reading

Apgar V, 1953. Proposal for a New Method of Evaluation of the Newborn Infant. (See above for more information.)

Montgomery K S, 2000. Apgar Scores : Examining the long-term significance. *Perinat. Educ.* 2000 Summer; 9(3): 5–9. doi: 10.1624/105812400X87716.Copyright. A Lamaze International Publication PMCID : PMC1595023. Available at: www.ncbi.nlm.nih.gov/pmc/articles/PMC1595023/

Oakley A, 1984. *The Captured Womb : A History of the Medical Care of Pregnant Women*. Oxford: Blackwell.

Odent M, 2002. *The Farmer and the Obstetrician*. London: Free Association Books.

Pert C, 1997. *Molecules of Emotion : Why You Feel the Way You Feel*. London: Simon and Schuster.

References

Apgar V, 1952/3. New York, N. Y. Department of Anesthesiology, Columbia University, College of Physicians and Surgeons and the Anesthesia Service, The Presbyterian Hospital. *Current Researches in Anesthesia and Analgesia*, July-August, 1953, p 260. Presented before the Twenty-Seventh Annual Congress of Anesthetists, Joint Meeting of the International Anesthesia Research Society and the International College of Anesthetists, Virginia Beach, Virginia, September 22-25, 1952. Website: www.placentalrespiration.net/Apgar.html

Clark DA, Hakanson DO, 1988. The inaccuracy of Apgar scoring Journal of Perinatology, Summer;8 (3) 203-5.

Department of Health, 1993. *Changing Childbirth*. London: HMSO.

Department of Health, 2007. *Maternity Matters*. London: HMSO.

Department of Health, 2004. *The National Service Framework for Children, Young People and Maternity Services*. London: HMSO.

Department of Health, 1992. *The Winterton Report*. House of Commons Health Select Committee. *Second Report on the Maternity Services*. London: HMSO.

Harrison M, 1993. A Woman in Residence. Ballantine Books.

Oakley A, 1986. The Captured Womb: A history of the medical care of pregnant women. Oxford: Blackwell.

Oakley A, 1980. *Women Confined : Towards a Sociology of Childbirth*. Oxford: Martin Robertson.

Odent M, 2002. *The Farmer and the Obstetrician*. London: Free Association Books

O'Donnell CP, Kamlin CO, Davis PG, Carlin JB, Morley CJ, 2006. Interobserver variability of the 5-minute Apgar score. *J Pediatr*, Oct;149(4):486-9.

4: Alienation and efficiency in postmodern institutions

"I don't want to express alienation. It isn't what I feel. I'm interested in various kinds of passionate engagement. All my work says be serious, be passionate, wake up."

Susan Sontag (1933-2004), American novelist

LEAN, NOT MEAN... LESSONS FROM TOYOTA

Following the Fordism approach to car manufacturing and maternity care so as to maximise efficiency, we are now entering an era of 'lean' thinking which also comes from another car manufacturer: Toyota.

Toyota has a long history of priding themselves on their excellence in engineering, producing high-quality cars and they have become a thriving global business leader in the car manufacturing industry. This success has largely been thanks to William Edwards Deming's philosophy and management teachings outlined in his book *The Deming Management Method* (Mercury Business Books, 1992). Deming believed that when people focus on quality, costs fall over time (measuring quality as being the results of work efforts divided by the total cost). This is because waste is reduced when services or products are produced that work better simply because there is less reworking required, greater staff loyalty, greater *customer* loyalty and less litigation. In manufacturing, the advantage of focusing on quality so as to engineer a long-term reduction in cost seems understandable as quality will clearly affect market share, productivity and profit over the longer term. In health care, this theory is less useful because quality is only aimed for so as to reduce *costs* (not to improve outcomes overall) but Deming's theory is nevertheless a likely cause of the outcome-driven metrics now being asked for in the NHS to monitor quality (DH, 2010). It is a theory which focuses on minimising costs while also emphasising quality, which makes it attractive and marketable to healthcare managers.

The first real sign of lean thinking seeping into the NHS became visible just over 10 years ago in the NHS Plan (2000), whose aim was to ensure that the NHS did the right thing, at the right time, in the right place. On the current NHS Innovations Institute (NHSII) website, this is now referred to as being a 'lean' ideology, which means doing the 'right things in the right place, at the right time, in the right quantities, while minimising waste and being flexible and open to change' (NHS II, 2010). Whilst this mirrors the aspirations of almost every doctor, midwife and other NHS employee, it is interesting that 10 years of discussions have taken place on lean thinking are still ongoing and that lean thinking is still seen as a relatively new way of thinking today. A key underpinning element is the need to involve and motivate staff in identifying the changes to be made and signing up to them. This is a great strength because once consensus has been achieved on a given issue, change is likely to be sustainable. The key principles of LEAN according to the NHSII in 2010 include:

- improving flow to eliminate waste and reduce delays
- getting things right first time, thus improving quality and lowering costs
- empowering staff and motivating them to sustain results
- making good decisions using evidence
- learning by doing so as to get results quickly

QUALITY—MORE IMPORTANT THAN PROCESS

Introducing lean thinking in the NHS is seen as a panacea for what is believed by many, including some very senior people, to be a confused, chaotic, disorganised and wasteful culture. Prime Minister David Cameron's description of the NHS as 'second rate' during a BBC Radio 4 *Today* programme whilst announcing his plans for the largest restructure the NHS has ever seen, caused a political uproar in January, 2010. It is worth noting that the shake-up he was announcing introduces competition and maintains inspection which, as will be discussed later in this chapter, goes against Deming's management teachings, which underpin Toyota's successes.

'Lean' assumes that by streamlining processes, we can reduce waste and thus increase quality, whilst reducing costs at the same time. There is no doubt that improving processes by involving those directly delivering care can both reduce waste and increase quality. One example of this has been the streamlining of the antenatal pathway enabling more women to have access to antenatal care early on in their pregnancies. The Care Quality Commission Survey in 2010 showed that over half of women had a booking appointment before 9 weeks and that 95% of women had an early dating scan, in line with best practice. In 2007, only 85% of women had an early dating scan so this is a significant improvement.

Another lean innovation which many women value is the development of 'one-stop antenatal screening clinics'. In this model, women are seen by a midwife before they attend the antenatal screening appointment. A full medical and obstetric history is taken and appropriate dietary and pregnancy advice given, including a discussion of antenatal screening. The women are then invited to attend an antenatal screening appointment before 12 weeks and 6 days gestation. During the appointment they have a blood test and nuchal ultrasound scan to screen for markers for chromosomal abnormality, particularly Down's syndrome. If the results suggest that a woman is at a higher risk of having a baby with a chromosomal abnormality, she is offered a chorionic villus sampling test and this can be carried out on the same day if she wishes. Of course, this is preferable to her having to endure an anxious wait of at least a couple of days and having to return for another appointment should the initial results suggest she is high risk. Therefore, by streamlining processes we can certainly improve women's pathways through care and reduce costs through reductions in extra appointment times and concomitant administration costs.

However, if we allow ourselves to become overly process-driven and only focus on cutting costs, there is a danger that we may reduce quality. Real quality care with minimal waste occurs in a maternity service where there are real relationships between women, midwives and the wider multidisciplinary and multi-agency team. Deming himself highlighted the link between quality and personal relationships between employees, suppliers and customers. In health care it is precisely when fragmentation of care occurs that most costs and risks escalate, however efficient the pathway looks on paper. Examples of this include tests being repeated needlessly because the person ordering them did not know they had already been done before, or worse still, results not being followed up appropriately or in a timely manner, thus requiring more intervention as a woman's condition becomes more complicated.

RELATIONSHIPS—THE KEY TO QUALITY

In the delivery of maternity care, the focus on improving quality of care will always be predominantly about the people themselves, what they value, what they believe, how they behave and how they interact. The systems and processes are an adjunct to this. Even in the car manufacturing industry, as we've seen, these 'softer' elements are important, but in maternity care they are vitally important if we are to prevent fragmentation and alienation of the people we are supposed to be caring for. If a system is purely process-driven, it's likely these softer elements will only occur by chance.

In fact, in my experience, it is often in the case of women with more complex medical, obstetric or psychosocial needs that fragmentation and duplication occur. It is still sometimes difficult for large organisations to be able to streamline the care of these women so that they can see the multi-disciplinary team at one appointment. However, even though, increasingly, maternity services are establishing joint clinics for women with diabetes, epilepsy or complex mental health needs, it seems that women who are most vulnerable are least likely to get the streamlined care which would most benefit them and the maternity services, by reducing waste. Indeed, it is now a widely accepted doctrine in the UK that every pregnant woman needs a midwife, and that having a midwives makes the process of childbirth better for both mother and baby. (Midwifery 2020: Delivering Expectations, 2010 certainly supports this view). It is this commitment to linking every woman to a midwife who sits at the hub of the maternity network which is most likely to deliver the best quality care for women and babies.

Therefore, while the introduction of lean thinking may be of benefit, it must not be used in isolation, treating women as a product which needs to be processed, because quality in health care involves much more than a series of processes. How quality is perceived depends on the direct impact healthcare provision has on women and their families.

The fact that fewer interventions are necessary for women receiving midwifery-led care and that outcomes are better (Hatem, 2009) underline how important it is for women to receive midwifery-led care with a small group of midwives. This is one obvious example to illustrate the importance of relationships on professional behaviours which are difficult to quantify under traditional lean thinking. In Hatem's study an analysis of 11 trials including

12,276 women showed that women receiving midwifery-led care were less likely to be admitted to hospital antenatally, have an epidural in labour, be given an episiotomy or have an operative vaginal birth. These women were also more likely to have a spontaneous birth without the use of pharmacological analgesia and to feel in control during their labour and birth. More mystifying but significant is the fact that these women were also less likely to experience fetal loss before 24 weeks gestation.

When women receive midwifery-led care from a small group of midwives the result is a whole range of improved outcomes

Another salient warning to those endeavouring to introduce quality care using lean principles without taking account of relationship dynamics is provided by Toyota itself. Disaster struck in 2010 when they had to recall millions of cars across the world because of a suspected design fault causing the accelerator to stick, and consequent car crashes, some of which caused fatalities. Toyota lost millions of pounds and a great deal of its market share across the world. Following this episode, some people criticised the working culture at Toyota and in Japan for being overly respectful of authority, arguing that this working culture made it difficult for employees to speak up, even though the systems to do so were in place.

The same phenomenon is often also seen in the field of health care when there is a perception of a very strong hierarchy. Perhaps this may, in part, have been the problem in Mid Staffordshire, where many elderly people suffered and died because of cuts in staffing and overcrowded wards. Interestingly, according to Haddon-Cave (2009) the same problem is a consistent theme across all major disasters, including the loss of the Nimrod XV230 aircraft, the loss of the space shuttles *Challenger* and *Columbia*, the capsizing of the Townsend Thoresen ferry *The Herald of Free Enterprise*, the King's Cross fire, the sinking of the pleasure boat the *Marchioness*, and the BP oil disaster of 2010. Cost cutting, strong personalities, pressurised work environments with tight deadlines and a steady trend of corner cutting mesh together to create a fearful working environment. In those situations even when systems are in place for raising concerns, these are often either not raised in the first place, or not taken seriously.

In pressurised work situations, concerns are often not raised

THE INADEQUACIES OF EXTERNAL VALIDATION

Currently there is still a heavy emphasis on inspection in health care so as to ensure quality. The badging and quality markers of success are used as a proxy for quality services. Yet these inspections often involve no more than a paper exercise. Arguably, 'Investors in people' initiatives and the NHSLA Clinical Negligence Scheme for ensuring Trust standards (see 'Further reading' at the end of this chapter) have done little in reality to ensure that quality care is provided, even though they have cost a great deal of money to achieve. In addition, if the government's intentions are to be believed, competition will be rife within the NHS and external validation and charter marks may become even more important as different organisations compete for business and the best staff at the expense of collaboration. Instead of these external attempts at validation, what is needed so as to ensure quality is intrinsic motivation of healthcare professionals. This would do far more to improve standards, outcomes and costs.

If the scandal at Mid Staffordshire Foundation Trust has taught the healthcare profession anything about quality and standards of care, it is that the industrial paper models of measurement and inspection fail miserably when it comes to delivering compassion, well-being, humanity and meaningful life. It should also teach us that 'lean' is great while quality of care remains the focus. However, if finance, productivity or the aspiration to be seen to achieve is the primary focus, there is a temptation to continually cut processes even though history tells us this will ultimately be at best counterproductive and at worst deleterious to health outcomes. In 2004 Liz Stephens recommended that we move to a whole new model of 'with woman' midwifery care; in her view the evidence suggests that many midwives are currently working more in a 'with institution' model. Relying on external validation from whatever source within the institution—from work colleagues, through paper exercises, inspection visits or league tables—can only be disempowering for women, midwives and other healthcare professionals, because it will mean that they are not truly 'with woman' during each woman's childbearing process. As long as we seek to achieve some man-made status symbol we are likely to be expending efforts needlessly... What is essential to quality care is an inner sense of personal commitment to excellence.

Many student midwives start their midwifery training as mature students, so they are women who have a lot of life experience, who have also often had children themselves. These women, and some men, come into the midwifery profession profoundly moved to give something back and yet often they very quickly become disillusioned with the gap between their aspirations and the working reality they experience. Qualified midwives also become disillusioned with their working reality (Curtis et al, 2006). What really perpetuates this gap between aspiration and reality? It is easy to blame lack of resources such as staffing levels, lack of equipment and stressful working environments but it goes deeper than that… I have worked in the NHS for over 30 years in many different hospitals at many different levels. What I have learnt from this experience is that whilst resources are important to quality care, the provision of sensitive maternity care is at least as much dependent on the values, attitudes and behaviour of the people delivering the service as on the resources themselves. In overly medicalised environments, resources may be squandered on unnecessary and sometimes invasive tests which, rather than adding to quality care, actually detract from it. As a result, midwives may become disempowered. Our professional reliance on external validation has led many midwives to have a small voice and become overwhelmed by the challenges ahead, to become subsumed in bureaucracy.

In addition, an overly process-orientated organisation which everyone is expected to follow rigidly can cause paralysis in individual decision-making because of the copious policies and guidelines which such a process-orientated system involves. Both policies and the pressure to follow them can detract midwives from engaging in useful, care-enhancing critical thinking.

The problem we now have, though, is that attitudes are changing in midwifery and society's expectations are also changing rapidly. What has worked before may not be appropriate for the future, particularly since women are now more aware that they want choice, continuity, control, better birth environments, birth in midwifery-led units and the option of home birth—and a life-enhancing experience generally in childbirth. Our professional reliance on bureaucracy has resulted in many midwives being simply engulfed by procedures.

> What has worked before may not be appropriate for the future, particularly since women are now more aware of what they want

Deming argued that to deliver real quality, it is important to move away from an inspection approach to ensuring quality. Instead, it is important to engage and inspire individuals from the Board right down to those directly on the manufacturing line, so as to sign all staff up to delivering the highest quality work they can manage, simply because they are proud of what they do and what the company stands for. Deming also advocated collaboration and co-operation over competition. Intrinsic motivation such as this is endemic in the NHS in the best possible sense, and it is arguably its greatest strength.

If we are to engage and inspire individuals within maternity services and really harness and develop any existing intrinsic motivation in this post-modern era, we need to re-establish internal values and work towards validation of a different kind, which comes partly from within. This is the internal validation that comes from a sense of a job well done; external validation can come at least partly from the women and babies we care for. Perhaps this idea is surprising to you... particularly if you are keenly aware of how colleagues have in the past turned on each other, as if in fierce professional and hierarchical competition. Instead of continuing to behave in this way we need to unite behind our common goal, which is to provide quality care for pregnant and labouring women, and new mothers. By working collaboratively with all our maternity care colleagues, we could positively transform the care women receive and also develop a real pride in our work and our profession.

In time, it is possible that lean thinking and the recession might provide a cathartic moment for maternity services, which may never come again. Medicalisation is costly and women's expectations are rightly increasing. Midwifery-led care, birth centres and the promotion of home birth are the keys to promoting normality. Promoting normality underpins much of the government's rhetoric and policy at the moment and it is the foundation stone of the National Service Framework for Maternity Services (2004), Maternity Matters (2007) and Midwifery 2020 (2010). In some spheres, including the powerful media, the shift to midwifery-led care which more 'normality' will necessarily involve is sometimes portrayed as a 'poison apple' or there is the implication that this will mean a second rate service. This is why there was a public outcry when it was suggested that some small and non-viable obstetric units should be turned into midwifery-led units. Rather than portraying this as an appropriate metamorphosis of resources, i.e. lean thinking at it's best, the media portrayed this proposed change as a way of 'downgrading' maternity services.

In conclusion, while it is clear that it is important for all professions engaged in maternity care, especially midwives, to opt for some lean thinking, it is also important for midwifery-led units not to be portrayed negatively as poison apples. Instead, they need to be portrayed as jewels in the crown of the NHS— as a means to improving and streamlining maternity care, so that the limited money available is spent appropriately so as to guarantee high quality care for all women. With the right woman in the right place at the right time, delivering evidence-based care and reducing overprocessing in true lean style will increase quality and reduce waste. The intrinsic motivation which will result among maternity care professionals will also result in an increase in efficiency and an overall improvement in outcomes.

In the next chapter I shall consider how language helps maternity care professional to exert power and influence change in political terms.

Exercises

1 What are the advantages of applying lean thinking in health care?

2 Which one thing might you stop doing if you were to apply lean thinking?

3 In your view, what would be the most important benefit of successfully stopping doing this one thing that you do only because of lean thinking?

4 Would there be any potential risks of stopping doing this thing?

5 What factors might stop you from changing your current practice?

Further reading

Clinical Negligence Scheme for Trusts. Available at: www.nhsla.com/Claims/Schemes/CNST

Department of Health, 2007. Making it better for mother and baby. London: HMSO.

Department of Health, 2007. Maternity Matters. London: HMSO.

National Institute for Innovation and Improvement, 2010. Lean thinking. Available at: www.institute.nhs.uk/building_capability/general/lean_thinking.html

Department of Health, 2004. The National Service Framework for Children, Young People and Maternity Module 11. London: HMSO.

Investors in People Award. Available at: www.investorsinpeople.co.uk

Porter AP, 2011. David Cameron denies he believes NHS is 'second rate'. Political Editor, *The Telegraph*, London, 17 Jan.

References

Curtis P, Ball L, Kirkham M, 2006. Why do midwives leave? (Not) being the kind of midwife you want to be. *British Journal of Midwifery*, 14(1), 27-31.

Deming WE, 1992. *The Deming Management Method.* New York: Mercury Business Books. (New ed. Originally published by Perigree Books in 1986.)

Department of Health, 2000. The NHS Plan. A plan for investment, a plan for reform. London: HMSO.

Department of Health, London, 2004. The National Service Framework for Children, Young People and Maternity Module 11. London: HMSO.

Department of Health, 2007. Maternity Matters. London: HMSO.

Department of Health, 2010. The NHS Outcomes Framework. London: HMSO.

Haddon-Cave C, 2009. The Nimrod Review An independent review into the broader issues surrounding the loss of the RAF Nimrod MR2 Aircraft XV230 in Afghanistan in 2006. 28 October. London: HMSO.

Hatem M, Sandall J, Devane D, Soltani H, Gates S, 2008. Midwife-led versus other models of care for childbearing women. *Cochrane Database of Systematic Reviews*, Issue 4. Art. No.: CD004667. DOI: 10.1002/14651858.CD004667.pub2

Midwifery Working Group, 2010. Report: *Midwifery 2020: Delivering expectations*. London. Website: www.midwifery2020.org

National Institute for Innovation and Improvement, 2010. *Lean Thinking.* Website: www.institute.nhs.uk/building_capability/general/lean_thinking.html

Porter AP, 2011. David Cameron denies he believes NHS is 'second rate'. Political Editor, *The Telegraph*, London, 17 Jan.

Stephens L, Pregnancy In Stewart M (eds), 2004. *Pregnancy, Birth and Maternity Care: Feminist Perspectives*. Edinburgh: Books for Midwives.

5: The politics and power of language

"Everything can change, but not the language that we carry inside us, like a world more exclusive and final than one's mother's womb."

Italo Calvino (1923-1985), Italian journalist and writer

Building on all that has gone before, particularly the discussion about reductionist thinking and the production-line model of maternity care, this chapter examines the politics and power of language as it is played out in maternity care. In Hans Christian Anderson's classic tale, *The Emperor's New Clothes*, everyone knew that the emperor was naked but they were all too afraid to tell him that he was duped into believing that he was wearing the finest clothing. This tale illustrates the duplicitous power of subservience to authority and how it can prevent individuals from speaking their own truth for fear that they are too stupid to voice an opinion or that their opinion will not be well received. I want to use this analogy to discuss how we defer to medical authority because we are afraid of challenging what we know to be untrue. I will also discuss how we use language as a cloak to desensitise ourselves and dress up our delusions over the way childbirth is being managed in our society.

FROM 'DELIVERY' TO 'BIRTH'

I don't believe it's any coincidence that in my attempts to change the use of the term 'delivery' to 'birth' on labour wards, I have often met with heavy resistance from doctors and also, surprisingly, from some midwives. I have been laughed at and ridiculed, and have even experienced outright aggression. I have been told that it does not matter which words we use and that I am wasting my time. I have also been forbidden from pursuing the change in terminology by some consultant obstetricians. On one 'delivery suite', the midwifery staff changed the word from 'birth' to 'birthing' and then used analogies of boats docking to mock and detract from the essence of what was happening during births. However, if the change in language is such an irrelevance, why does it create such turmoil? Through language we communicate concepts, ideas and ideology (Thornton, 1998). Our language conveys social meaning and expected norms. So why is it that 'delivery' has become the norm for birth?

As a child grows, we don't celebrate his or her 'delivery day', we celebrate his or her 'birthday' as the anniversary of a unique and very special milestone in his or her life. In many cultures in the world, this tradition lasts throughout a person's lifetime. Curiously, there does not seem to be the same issues of sterile control of language used at the other end of life. The words 'death' and 'dying' are finite in their definitions and, unlike the word 'delivery', they do not share alternative meanings. As well as meaning the transference of a package from one place to another, delivery also means 'rescue' and 'relief' and the word therefore has the connotation of 'saving' women from childbirth. Delivery can also be made into a verb—'deliver'—and when used in the passive form it conveys a sense of an action taken, of a job done and of an episode finished. So once the woman is 'delivered', there is a strong sense that the medical profession has done its job.

The concept of 'delivery'—with all the connotations I've described—is deeply ingrained in many labour ward cultures and its appearance on the white board common to almost all labour wards where crucial details of women's progress in labour is logged seems appropriate, given the way in which it's used. This board is the backbone of most labour wards and it acts as the 'command centre' of the shift. The word 'delivered' or 'del' (a midwifery customised abbreviation) is written against the woman's name as soon as midwives or doctors become aware that the baby is born, often even before the placenta has been expelled. The alternative of writing 'baby born' or 'born' is virtually never used.

Unlike the word 'delivery', the word 'birth' has connotations of starting, not ending... of new beginnings, so the word 'delivery' is the 'sunset' which fits the curative medical model of birth, because it indicates that something has been completed. (This will be discussed in greater depth in Chapter 12.) However, a birth is the dawn of a new beginning; it indicates new life and a fresh start, all of which are mysteriously future-focused and which cannot be quantified. Thus, the use of the word 'birth' would embed the notion of the continuum of life inherent in a social model of midwifery.

'DELIVERY' AND OWNERSHIP OF BIRTH

Midwives often speak of having 'just had a delivery' but 'delivery' in this case is not a concrete noun (as in a parcel), so what is it they've had exactly? They may have witnessed another woman's birth experience but they have not had a baby because the baby belongs to the mother. If the midwife were to say 'I have just had a baby' that would sound ludicrous because everyone would know that the midwife had not just given birth. It is interesting to note that, when using this phrasing, the baby remains an individual—a person in its own right—and the mother's role in childbirth is not usurped by that of the doctor or midwife. Treating abstract nouns like 'delivery' as if they were concrete means that healthcare professionals are actually using language without meaning. Interestingly and paradoxically, though, the word 'delivery' does communicate strong abstract connotations of ownership, institutionalisation and medicalisation.

Another example of the use of abstract nouns as concrete nouns occurs in the case of the word 'education'. Politicians often talk about 'delivering education' but 'to educate' is a verb. The odd use of verbs in this way allows for deep generalisations to be made and for uncomfortable questions to remain hidden. In the case of the word 'delivery' when applied to childbirth, using the word hides the sexual nature of birth, the raw uncertainty of life and the moment of awareness of the fragility of humanity. In fact, sterile conversations which use the words 'delivery' and 'delivered' fill our maternity hospitals. As a result, those deeper emotional aspects of birth can become less important than physical ritual and routines which can start to dominate care, such as weighing, labelling and dressing the baby. These rituals and routines, protected by our language, can start to take precedence over intimate and essential skin-to-skin contact between mother and baby. Once ritual and routine dominate, any chance of maximising benefit for mother and baby, of helping them to treasure the first few moments together following birth, are lost forever.

Some people may argue that the words 'delivery' and 'delivered' are used simply to convey the end of labour but, as I mentioned before, in fact these words are often used when the placenta is still in situ or when the woman is having a postpartum haemorrhage. It is therefore clearly not being used to mean the end of labour because this is usually defined as the time after the complete delivery of the placenta and membranes, or (in some definitions) as the time after any excess bleeding has been controlled.

In fact, the words 'delivery' and 'delivered' are used to stop midwives and doctors from facing the raw reality of the emotional event that childbirth is. The depersonalisation that the word 'delivery' conveys, makes it easier to accept the often intimate and potentially degrading activities which happen daily on labour wards, such as the use of lithotomy position, vaginal examinations, fetal blood sampling, internal monitoring and rectal examinations, to name but a few. It is more to our shame that many of these intimate interventions are used too frequently and sometimes unnecessarily even today. For instance, the Care Quality Commission Survey (2010) showed a significant increase in the number of women giving birth in lithotomy (stirrups), with 30% of women giving birth in the lithotomy position, compared to 27% in 2007. Of the 30% of women who gave birth in the lithotomy position, only 14% had an instrumental birth. Therefore, a significant 16% of women gave birth 'normally' in the lithotomy position, even though lithotomy is traditionally only used for instrumental births. When the position is associated with normal birth, it is necessary to question whether midwives are choosing to put women in this position in the second stage, perhaps in the mistaken belief that doing so will aid pushing—even though there is absolutely no evidence to support this, given that lithotomy is a supine position. Indeed, the NICE intrapartum care guideline states that supine positions are associated with more pain, fetal heart rate anomalies and an increase in the rate of instrumental births (NICE, 2008). In addition, there are other side effects associated with lithotomy, such as the sustaining of nerve damage resulting in foot drop. Gottvall et al (1995) who studied 12,782 women who'd had a spontaneous vaginal birth identified that women in lithotomy had double the risk of anal sphincter tears. It is highly unlikely that women are requesting to give birth in the degrading lithotomy position so this must again be an example of midwives' control over women during labour and of their desensitisation to the fact that lithotomy is degrading. In fact, is even more degrading when you factor in that the beds in rooms on labour wards usually face towards the door, leaving women highly exposed, should someone enter the room.

Desensitisation is a protective measure that enables midwives and doctors to continue to work in a system which is detrimental to the well-being of women and their newborn babies. If it were not for desensitisation, their own inner dissonance would be so strong that midwives and doctors would have to strive to change the system or decide to leave the profession. For some people working in these professions, it is precisely the realisation of this dissonance that makes them leave. However, rather than shy away from this dissonance, we need to embrace it, for it is only when we begin to feel uncomfortable working in our current maternity care environments that we will be able to generate the change necessary to restore birth to a more respectful space. If we were to use the words 'birth' or 'baby born', we might be encouraged to engage our sense of self and our sense of celebration. This would interrupt at a subconscious level our desensitisation processes, which shield us from these uncomfortable truths.

> We need to embrace any dissonance we might feel and generate the change necessary to restore birth to a more respectful space

I have heard a 'ventouse delivery' being justified because the labour ward was getting busy and it was felt safest to undertake the procedure in good time. (If more time had been given to the woman to try and facilitate a normal birth, perhaps it would have been more difficult in terms of staffing.) The intervention in this woman's case was therefore driven purely by the needs of the institution... I don't believe this would happen if we, as healthcare professionals, held birth as sacrosanct. If we honoured birth, I believe we would find it much easier to move from the 'just in case' towards an 'Is it really necessary?' philosophy as regards medical intervention. History gives plenty of examples of procedures that the medical profession has carried out which have proven to be unnecessary and sometimes even harmful. It is easier to recognise older fallacies that have fallen by the wayside in previous generations such as leeches, bloodletting, routine hysterectomy, frontal lobotomy, shaving women prior to birth, administering enemas prior to birth and routine episiotomy—but it is much harder to explore what is unnecessary in present-day practices. The indiscriminate use of CTG persists in some areas despite the evidence widely known in the UK since 2001 when the first NICE guideline on fetal monitoring was released. There are other cases too... What about insertion of cannula in the case of women who have had more than four babies, performing an episiotomy for a 'rigid perineum' (which is most often simply failure to wait), the practice of using the lithotomy position for normal birth, or the performance of excessive vaginal examinations? What is of serious concern is that it is largely midwives, the guardians of normality, who are the administrators of these interventions.

> What is of serious concern is that it is largely midwives, the guardians of normality, who are the administrators of these interventions...

On a trip to the Middle East in 2007 I was surprised to learn that midwives were still carrying out routine perineal shaving and administering enemas to women in labour on admission as standard practice. These midwives had been trained in the UK, so they knew they were not carried out in Britain, and they also knew that neither of these practices were evidence-based. (The evidence showed that these were ineffective interventions and so wrong.) During one discussion, the midwives wanted to know how they could stop this practice. To me the answer was simple: refuse to do it. (This would be effective because doctors would not be prepared to carry out these procedures themselves.) Yet I realise now that on a deeper level, it's not so simple because these practices during childbirth reflect the disempowerment of women and midwives in society as a whole. The midwives were conforming because they were being controlled and because they were fearful of the consequences of not doing as they were instructed. The difficulties the midwives were describing in trying to stop giving routine enemas and shaves illustrated the degree of control being exerted, albeit often covertly. Although it's always easier to criticise another culture's culturally-driven behaviours because it's easier to see them for what they are, it's much harder to stand back and look at our own culturally-driven behaviours with the same objectivity. This is why paying attention to the language we use is crucial, as it can act as a lever for change.

In fact, the language used to describe the moment of birth is powerful because the word 'delivery' labels the woman a passive receptacle during birth, it also makes her baby a 'package, which is unceremoniously despatched. Therefore, by complying with the 'delivery' terminology, we are complicit in undermining the baby's welcome into the family and in undermining the baby's arrival we are letting down both women and their babies during childbirth.

OUR DELIVERY SUITE EMPIRES

Throughout the latter part of the last century, the word 'delivery' has also been busy empire-building. 'Delivery suite' is the term used for most modern labour wards and, once again, this is a term which depersonalises a momentous event and the people involved. Mass production is the nuance of the day. The phrase itself—'delivery suite'—creates a mental image of many rooms collectively placed around or very close to an operating theatre, each room having passive women awaiting help, so as to be relieved of their 'packages'. Over the last 27 years of my midwifery career, working in many different maternity services, I have collected photographs of 'delivery rooms' in many units.

58 welcoming baby

Surprisingly little has changed in that time, despite exhortations from women, The National Childbirth Trust, and national directives to make the rooms less clinical, more homely and woman-focused. It seems that we have managed to create a culture where homely environments are the speciality of birth centres and there is no need to create the same on labour wards. Across the world, from the United States, Australia and Abu Dhabi to the United Kingdom, the 'delivery rooms' in our hospitals are all equipped remarkably similarly. The 'delivery rooms' are easily identifiable, regardless of unit. The 'delivery' bed is always in the middle of the room, ostensibly so that staff can surround the woman on all sides at any time, should an emergency arise. Commonly, incontinence pads are placed in the middle of the bed over the top of the stark, white linen. And a hospital gown is placed on the bed ready for the woman to undress and give herself up to be 'delivered'.

Surprisingly little has changed, despite exhortations from women, The National Childbirth Trust, and national directives to make rooms less clinical, more homely and woman-focused

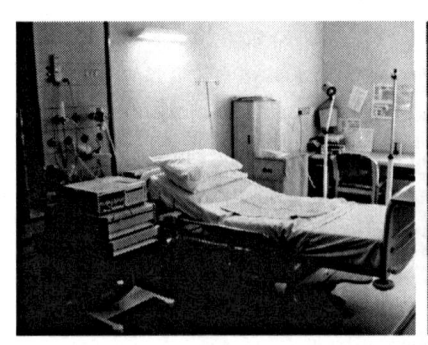

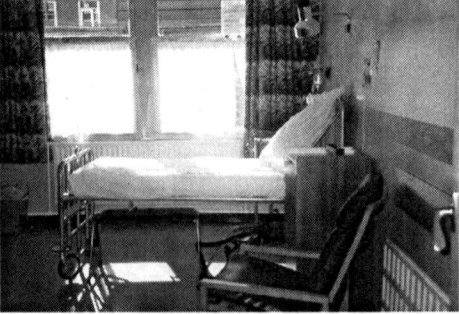

Above and below: A range of 'delivery' rooms I have seen... all remarkably similar

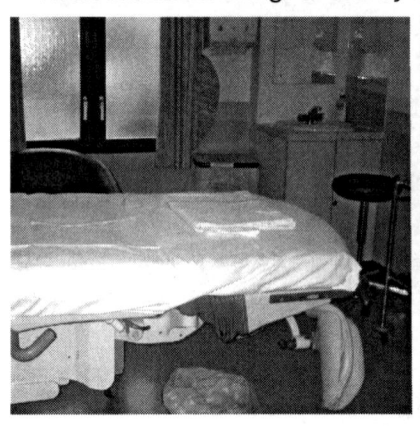

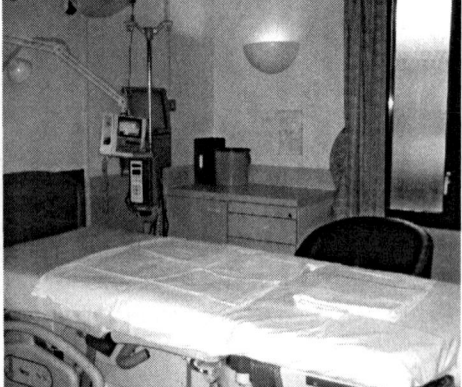

At one point in this new millennium, I worked in a hospital in London where the gowns provided so courteously to women were printed with the words 'hospital property' arranged in a pattern so as to deter people from stealing them. Thus the woman was totally subsumed in the hospital delivery suite culture and was indeed, for a period of time, even labelled 'hospital property.'

> The words 'hospital property' were arranged in a pattern on the hospital gown—so the woman was even labelled 'hospital property'

The reason for the hospital gown is to prevent women's own clothes from getting 'messy' during labour. Yet by encouraging women to adopt institutional clothing, we are immediately discarding another aspect of individuality which can make all the women look and seem the same, especially to the institutionally-focused staff. This is particularly poignant for some junior doctors on labour wards ('delivery suites') in the current system as the nature of their roles is that they tend to go from room to room dealing with different problems and can spend relatively little time actually getting to know the women. Since hospital gowns have to be used when an epidural is sited, inevitably on labour wards women start to look more and more similar so they end up all being treated the same.

Midwives may hopefully, given good staffing levels, be able to offer one-to-one care in labour and they may be more in a position to form a relationship with the women they care for. However, midwives have to actually be in the room with a woman, engaging in discussions in close proximity in order to support her. Greene's filmed documentary evidence of midwives and doctors in labour rooms caring for women in labour is fascinating (Greene, 2010). Some interludes of film depict supportive care, with the midwives engaging fully, while other interludes depict precisely the opposite. This makes it clear that although ensuring staffing levels are high enough to enable one-to-one midwifery care in labour is vital to quality care, it may not necessarily address all of the problems.

> Midwives have to actually be in the room with a woman, engaging in discussions in close proximity in order to support her—but even then some midwives may not engage fully

'WOMEN' OR 'PATIENTS'... DOES IT MATTER?

While we are talking about language, I would also like to comment on the use of the word 'patient' to describe women using maternity services. As an adjective the word 'patient' means 'being able to accept or tolerate delays, problems or suffering, without becoming annoyed or anxious' and the noun means 'registered to receive medical treatment or being in receipt of it' (according to the Oxford Dictionary at http://oxforddictionaries.com/definition/patient.) Combined, the two definitions conjure up an image of a passive woman registered to receive medical treatment or actually treatment. Yet women are healthy and pregnancy and childbirth are meant to be normal physiological processes, not phases of ill health—although, admittedly, some women do need medical treatment.

> The word 'patient' means 'being able to accept or tolerate delays, problems or suffering, without becoming annoyed or anxious' or 'registered to receive medical treatment or being in receipt of it'

The problem with calling women 'patients' is that it again desensitises the healthcare providers to the needs of the women they are caring for. There have recently been concerns about the importance of NHS staff treating 'patients' with compassion and as individuals at the point of care. It is interesting, in this respect, that the King's Fund Report into how to improve this softer aspect of care in the NHS is called 'Seeing the person in the patient' (Goodrich and Cornwell, 2008) and that the report says that delivering care compassionately goes beyond customer-care training.

When we call women 'patients' we are in essence using medical terminology which homogenises and suppresses the individuality of women's experience of childbirth and which confirms our acceptance that childbirth is a medical event.' For this reason, I believe the word 'patient' to be an inappropriate word to describe women receiving midwifery care during pregnancy and childbirth. The fact that some midwives continue to use the 'patient' terminology is a reminder of just how medicalised birth has become. In a survey asking women what they would prefer to be called, the outcome was that they would prefer to be called 'women' or 'mothers'. Clearly, even women are aware of the pitfalls of being labelled with a label which implies that they are in need of medical treatment. At least southern Ireland has got it right because they say that health care needs to be 'people-centred', not 'patient-centred'.

LANGUAGE UNDERPINS OUR THINKING

A woman's potential for having an empowering birth experience with her family is institutionally undermined when all attention is focused on delivering care on the 'delivery suite' 'efficiently' and 'effectively', with an emphasis on processing women as 'patients' in need of medical 'care' and 'delivery' from their condition of having a baby inside them. Depersonalised language underlines the process-driven approach and overshadows an element of birth which is unquantifiable and so often unrecognised in our rational, scientific world of maternity care. Language is powerful but because its power is unrecognised it is frequently given little consideration or attention.

Any new baby deserves to be welcomed gently and lovingly into the world. His or her birth is the start of a life journey and he or she deserves to have the best possible introduction to his mother, father and significant others, on whom he or she is going to be dependent for survival, physically, emotionally and psychologically. It is the start of the most significant and profound relationships which will probably continue throughout his or her lifetime.

Since life is not necessary easy and since it may not always go as anticipated for the baby or the parents, every scrap of psychological and emotional resource and resilience is needed within both parents and the child to help the life journey be a rewarding and positive experience. The use of language to camouflage the importance of the event of birth for both mother and baby and to enable mass baby-producing labour wards to thrive under the auspices of safety, must be reviewed. Healthcare professionals must make their use of terminology value individuality and personal autonomy and the celebration of birth and motherhood. When we do so, we will automatically significantly change the way in which we view our world of maternity care and we will improve how we deliver that service.

Already as I write this, I see there are the beginnings of change in language use in some national documents but change is slow, especially in terms of how staff interact with each other on a daily basis and in terms of how they interact with women and their families. It's time for us to talk about the Emperors' new clothes—i.e. the explicit influencing of attitudes and procedures through the use of language—which we see all around us. And instead of putting clothes on an emperor, in this case we need to acknowledge the power and politics of language and strip it out of our communication in any cases where it clouds our perceptions. We need to show these words up for what they are: a smoke and mirrors trick to convince people that what we are currently doing is not only right, but the only way to deliver maternity care. If we really are to generate sensitive birth practices, then ensuring we use appropriate language to convey what we mean is a good starting point... for the use of language can have far-reaching effects. After all, we must remember that it has been through the use and challenge of certain words that much discrimination has been first highlighted and then eliminated, and that behaviours have eventually been changed for the better.

> We need to show certain words up for what they are: a smoke and mirrors trick to convince people that what we are currently doing is not only right, but the only way to deliver maternity care

The next chapter stays with the theme of language and power and examines how they curiously inhabit the world of the hospital labour ward environment. I explore how power politics lie beneath maternity hospital design in a seemingly innocuous way.

Exercises

1 Keep a diary of how often the terms 'birth' and 'delivery' are used in conversations you participate in or overhear, in text books or novels, and in the media, etc, and note the source each time you notice it being used.

2 Using your diary for reflection, see if you can spot patterns and trends relating to the preference for the use of the word 'birth' over the word 'delivery, or 'delivery' over 'birth'.

3 Construct sentences reflecting the work that midwives and doctors do in facilitating birth without using the word 'delivery'.

4 If you work in maternity services commit to spending a whole day not using the word 'delivery' and reflect on the experience of doing so.

5 Reflect on what term you personally feel most comfortable using and analyse why.

Further reading

Bayar A, Keser S, Hosnuter M, Tanriverdi A, Ege A, 2007. Lower Limb Compartment Syndrome After an Uncomplicated Labor. *ORTHOPEDICS,* November 30 (11): 972.

Goodrich J, Cornwell J, 2008. Seeing the person in the patient. *The Point of Care review paper.* London: The King's Fund.

References

Care Quality Commission Survey into Maternity Services, Dec 2010. Website: www.cqc.org.uk/aboutcqc/howwedoit/involvingpeoplewhouseservices/patientsurveys/maternity_services.cfm

Goodrich J, Cornwell J, 2008. Seeing the Person in the Patient. London: The Kings Fund.

Gottvall K, Allebeck P, Ekeus C, 1995. Risk factors for anal sphincter tears: the importance of maternal position at birth. BJOG: *An International Journal of Obstetrics and Gynaecology* 114(10):1266-1272.

Greene K, 2010. Presentation at Advanced Labour Ward Practice. Royal College of Obstetricians and Gynaecologists, 1 March.

National Institute for Health and Clinical Excellence, 2008. Intrapartum Care. June. London: NICE. Website: www.NICE.org.uk

Thornton T, 1998. *Wittgenstein On Language and Thought. Philosophy of Content.* Edinburgh: Edinburgh University Press.

6: Patterns of power in the delivery suite

"The limits of my language are the limits of my mind. All I know is what I have words for."

Ludwig Wittgenstein (1889-1951), Austrian philosopher

LANGUAGE AS A SPYHOLE TO CORE VALUES

Language can be used as a spy hole to our core values. As discussed in the last chapter, the word 'delivery' has been helped us to build our empires. After 'delivery' became the preferred term for giving birth, 'delivery suite' became the preferred term used to describe most modern labour wards, although 'labour ward' is at least more honest. Women giving birth do indeed 'labour', unless they have an elective caesarean section, and since the time when childbirth moved into the hospital institution, that has usually happened within a hospital ward environment.

> *The birth of a baby is probably the closest anyone comes to their own immortality*

Interestingly the word 'labour' had 25 different definitions in the Oxford English dictionary in 1978, 10 of which refer to hard work and the physical or mental difficulties associated with it, with 6 of these including the concept of 'pain' within the definition. Even today, any definition of labour has an emphasis on hard physical or manual work. It seems that great effort, pain and a sense of achievement are synonymous with the majority of definitions of 'labour' and this mirrors the experience of many women during childbirth. The somewhat tenuous link with Hercules' labours and his quest for immortality is also pertinent in a spiritual way as each woman aspires to the birth of a live healthy baby. After all, the birth of a baby is probably the closest anyone comes to their own immortality (Gould, 2000).

The birth of a baby is probably the closest we come to immortality

Despite the enormity of birth, we subconsciously choose to use terminology in our busy maternity hospitals which circumvents any recognition of women's hard work and achievement in the production of their babies. The professional terminology concentrates attention on the moment the baby is 'delivered' and begs the question: delivered by whom? It also focuses attention on the end event rather than on the process of life's journey of discovery. It brings finality to the birth process while, in fact, from a lifetime perspective, it is only the beginning.

Indeed, following the 'delivery', the intense medical attention that women have received throughout their pregnancy and labour is almost immediately stopped, or at least abruptly diminished. This is evidenced by the fact that postnatal support has long been criticised as being the 'Cinderella' of maternity care, with many women wishing for more support to help them get used to caring for their baby and for more help with breastfeeding (Healthcare Commission, 2008, Care Quality Commission, 2010).

The authority imbued in the word 'delivery' and its ability to depersonalise and diminish the power and individual achievement of women during childbirth is clear. Yet its associations are further enhanced by the term 'delivery suite', particularly since the word 'suite' is not a term commonly used in everyday speech. It is a formal and somewhat twee term and it's astounding that it should come to be associated with such a powerful paradigm as labour and birth. Yet, at the same time, is its use indicative of what we as a society are trying to hide from?

The NICE intrapartum care guideline (2007) opens by reinforcing the fact that the majority of women having babies are healthy, with uncomplicated pregnancies, and should therefore be treated as normal. NICE also recommends that women should be told that having a baby in this country is very safe (NICE, 2007). It is interesting to contrast this recommendation with the seemingly contradictory messages women are receiving. The discussion below will reveal a very different subliminal effect the current institutionalisation of birth has on women's perception of risk.

Throughout the world, childbirth is defined and managed differently, according to how each culture interprets it. The most powerful members of any society define the interpretation and subsequent management of childbirth (Oakley, 1993, Kitzinger, 1992). In the UK maternity care is defined and controlled by the medical profession even when maternity care is delivered through a midwifery model. The gradual medicalisation of childbirth has occurred through the window of the abnormal/normal interface which separates midwifery from obstetrics. The tensions between this interface has historically been exploited by the medical profession to gain control over midwifery and thus move childbirth away from the domain of the midwife into the realms of the obstetric profession (Donnison, 1998). So while midwives often think of themselves as practitioners in their own right, it is in fact incongruous for them to do so when they are largely controlled by guidelines and protocols agreed and defined by obstetricians. Until midwives start to clearly define normal midwifery parameters and establish what their role is, they will continue to see their role eroded, despite rhetorical support of the role of the midwife from the medical profession and the government. The difficulty for midwives is that this power and control dynamic is being played out largely at a subconscious level in society at large. Lip service is also paid to the autonomous role of the midwife, but some midwives hesitate to rise to the challenge of accepting the responsibility and accountability that necessarily accompanies autonomous practice. Independent midwives are probably the midwives who come closest to embracing autonomy today.

OUR THOUGHTS ARE HOSTAGES TO LANGUAGE

NICE asserts that "All women in labour should be treated with respect and should be in control of and involved in what is happening to them, and the way in which care is given is key to this" (2007, p7).

In this respect the language we use, specifically the words, frame concepts and our belief in differing realities. Wittgenstein, a philosopher interested in language and thought, argued that we cannot possibly really know what another person is thinking and saying because so much information is lost in translation from thought through to expression of ideas during the process of communication. He also argued that it is language, or a lack of it, that limits thoughts of future possibilities (Thornton, 1998).

Professional communication, which is so dependent on language, is still an ongoing problem and our struggle to articulate the deleterious effects of certain practices in a meaningful way is evidence of this. Perhaps this is because, following Wittgenstein's line of thought, if we do not have a 'word' to identify something, it is as if it doesn't exist because we cannot actually communicate what it is to other people. In fact, some people would argue that there has henceforth been no need for the word to exist the new idea may be irrelevant in our society at a particular time.

Once something is acknowledged as a new concept in a culture, words usually emerge to describe it

Dictionaries do evolve over time, though, and new words are admitted to them as society changes. The Oxford English Dictionary updates words quarterly and such changes are obviously essential. One clear, recent, rather sinister addition to the dictionary was the word 'cyber bullying' which means to send threatening messages through emergent electronic communication systems (e.g. by email or text message, or via Facebook). So, clearly, once something is acknowledged as a new concept in a culture, words usually emerge to describe it. On this note, it is curious and interesting that different languages group concepts differently—for example different languages appear to have different numbers of words for 'love' because speakers of different languages like to refer to love in different ways. What does this say about the differences between societies and perhaps the interdependencies for survival which may play out in some places, where there is more of an emphasis on describing shades of love? In the UK, where we have relatively few words to describe love, we may be less focused on different types of love because we are more comfortable in our environment. This could be to our detriment as our illusion of physical comfort and protection may conceal inner emotional harm.

Even though words make up a proportion of communication, words remain incredibly powerful because they convey meaning and build concepts

Even though words make up a proportion of communication— body language and tone of voice being important adjuncts—words remain incredibly powerful because they convey meaning and build concepts. Even bureaucratic bodies such as NICE are becoming aware of the importance of the words we use. Advice from NICE includes the recommendation that all caregivers need to establish good rapport, and the way to do this, it is suggested, is to ask the woman about her wants and expectations for labour, and to be 'aware of the importance of tone and demeanour, and of the actual words they use" (NICE, 2007, p7). The suggestion is clearly that ideas are hostage to words and that they are important for communicating and interpreting meaning. This is why it is essential to explore further how we use them.

68 welcoming **baby**

'DELIVERY SUITE'—THE 'MATCHING SET' SYNDROME

The word 'suite' suggests 'a group', 'a matching set' or 'a collection'. Clearly, this is an accurate term used to describe a labour ward, given that any large labour ward will have a collection of rooms which are usually interconnected to allow access for healthcare professionals. Interestingly, the rooms are also usually identical in layout with similar decor and the cupboards all stocked with the same equipment and supplies so that staff know exactly where everything is. As I mentioned before, it is highly unusual to find anything different and 'delivery rooms' are easily identifiable, regardless of hospital.

As well as the individual delivery rooms being similar, what is remarkable is how similar layouts of the 'delivery suite' or 'labour ward' are, both old and new.

> It is highly unusual to find anything different.
> What is remarkable is how similar the layouts of
> the 'delivery suite' or 'labour ward' are, both old and new.

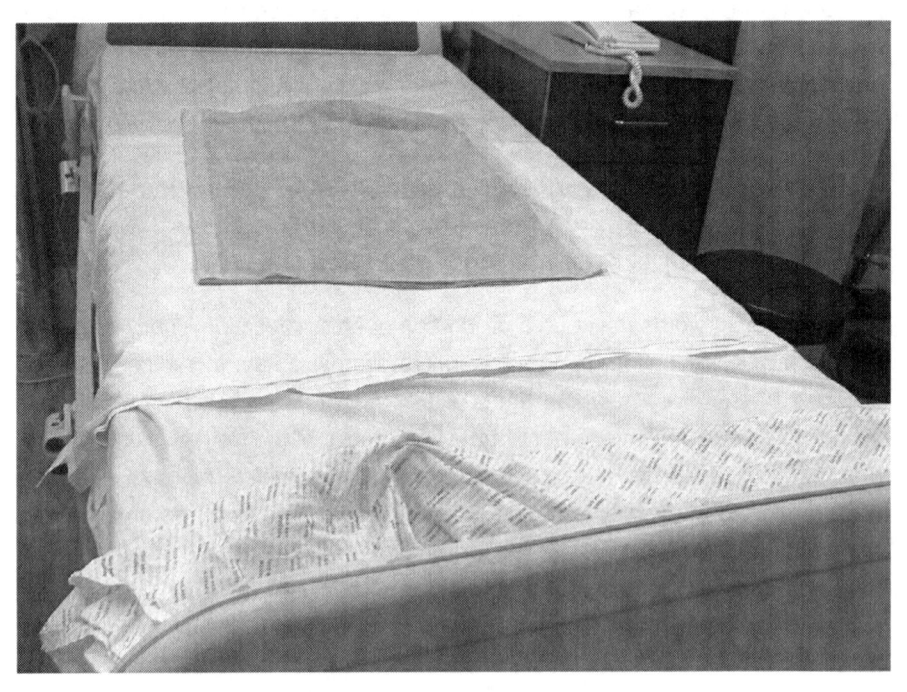

A bed with an incontinence pad 'ready' to soak up body fluid and a hospital gown so that the woman can undress and give herself up to be 'delivered'

6: Patterns of power in the delivery suite 69

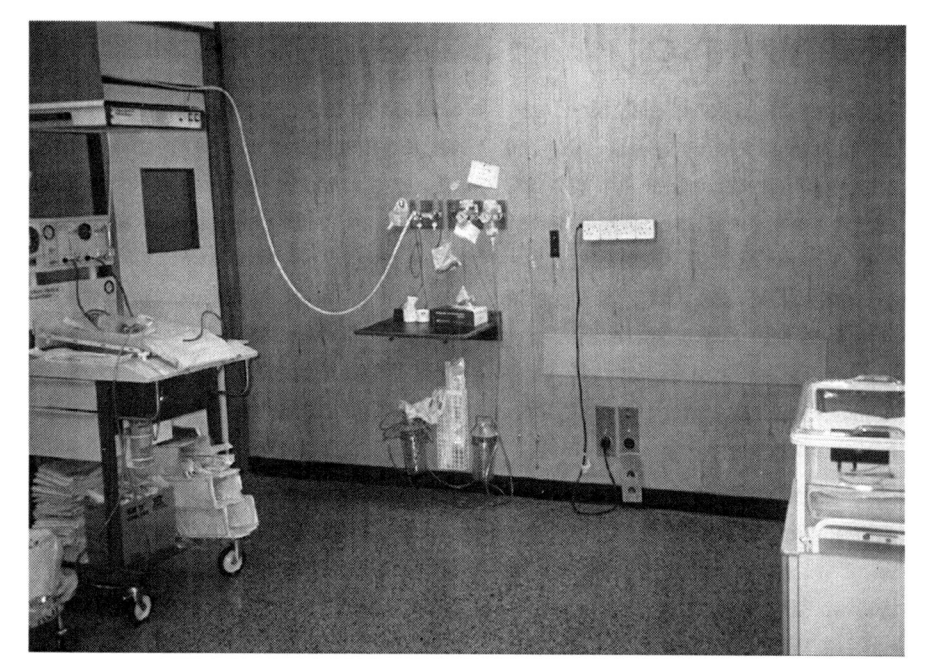

A photo of a second stage room in 1984, a time when women were moved to a different, theatre-like room to give birth

Architects over time seem to have come to the conclusion that a race-track style works best. As already discussed, this is translated into an image of many rooms collectively placed around or very close to an obstetric operating theatre (as outlined in Safer Childbirth, 2007). In the UK, this means we can usually undertake an emergency caesarean section in less than 30 minutes, should a Category 1 caesarean section be required, because there are life-threatening circumstances to mother or baby (NICE, 2004). Being very close to the operating theatre now seems normal, and indeed comforting, for doctors and midwives. This is also, increasingly, becoming a source of comfort for many women and their families in our society, as the complications associated with childbirth are amplified in the media to the detriment of the perception of the safety of normal childbirth in healthy women with uncomplicated pregnancies.

> The complications associated with childbirth are amplified in the media to the detriment of the perception of the safety

THE IMPACT OF PROFESSIONAL PREFERENCES

Professional power is also significant in relation to the design of new maternity units. Many of the newest maternity units are designed with furnishings and fittings which mean that you can *only* put the bed in the middle of the room. The rooms are large but seldom large enough to conceal equipment that is available 'just in case' and so much of it stays on show, particularly the resuscitaires used to resuscitate the baby, if required. These are large pieces of equipment complete with overhead heater, oxygen and air cylinders and all the equipment for intubation and advanced resuscitation. This resuscitation equipment is familiar and reassuring to staff, yet perhaps a little frightening to many women and their partners.

It is difficult to promote normality and reassurance that all is well when women are labouring alongside a machine designed for resuscitation of their baby. Yet in our current society we are so indoctrinated to regard this as 'normal', that we stop seeing it. This is partly because labour rooms and maternity units have a large input in their design by the staff working in existing hospitals. Hence, a large part of the building is designed to suit their needs, not necessarily those of the women and families who will be using them. Many of the staff involved will have trained for many years in the fields of medicine—perhaps in midwifery or nursing, or in other professions allied to health. Thus, many of the people consulted about the design of any new facilities would have spent the majority of their adult working lives in hospitals so, for them, the hospital environment seems familiar and safe.

Humans have an ability to adapt to changing surroundings over time, whatever they may be. Inevitably this adaptation takes us through stages of fear or apprehension, habituation and familiarity, then ultimately a comfort zone forms. Given this psychological background to those having a strong voice in designing hospitals, it is no wonder that little has changed in their layouts over the decades. Also, the design helps allay healthcare workers' personal fears about not being able to cope in acute emergency situations, and satisfying this need often happens at the expense of focusing on the needs of the woman for the majority of the time. This again illustrates the rescuer-victim modality which is subconsciously factored into every labour ward design, where the focus remains almost entirely on dealing with medical emergencies.

Professional dominances and allegiances can also be observed when new maternity units are being designed and decisions made often reflect dominant preferences. Inevitably, in a new building compromises will have been made relating to where different interdependent and allied services are placed, because it is highly unusual to have enough space for everything to be on one floor. This means that if floors are to be designed from scratch, a decision needs to be made as to whether the labour ward is placed with the neonatal intensive care unit alongside it, or whether it is positioned alongside postnatal rooms with neonatal care... The alignments chosen vary around the country from maternity unit to maternity unit and this in itself indicates that there is no professional consensus on what constitutes a priority alliance.

The fact that some variation exists in preferred co-locations suggests that the choices are, in fact, culturally driven, despite being portrayed as clinically required. Thus the design can reveal the sometimes covert beliefs, preferences and power dynamics of the clinical professionals involved in the design team. For instance, if you have a neonatal unit on the same floor as the labour ward, this arrangement is clearly seen as being clinically best for the woman and her baby—no doubt because there is quick and easy access to the neonatal unit, should it be required at birth. Nevertheless, it is the labour ward and neonatal staff who largely benefit from easy access between the two, making their working lives smoother because they do not have to walk too far between areas. After all, a new mother who has had a premature baby, or who is unwell (perhaps because she has had a difficult birth or a caesarean section) will not benefit from the same arrangement... Several times in any 24-hour period she will need to make her way to a different area, which is possibly even on a different floor simply so as to visit her new baby. This is because the decision to co-locate the labour ward and neonatal services effectively displaces postnatal care and therefore also the mother. At present, rarely are neonatal units aligned with postnatal wards in our institutions, although there are some maternity units with this configuration. Furthermore, almost never are new mothers routinely cared for in the vicinity of neonatal units, even when their babies are very sick. There are usually some family rooms to use if a baby is very sick or if he is almost ready for discharge and breastfeeding needs to be further established, but hospital design does not really encapsulate women and their families as the centre of care; design is still professionally driven.

Coming back to the terminology used—to the phrase 'delivery suite'—we should note that the term 'suite' is usually associated with the word 'set'—and in this sense we usually find ourselves thinking of tea sets, lounge furniture and bathroom fittings.

In fact, women in labour are also a 'matching set' of sorts. Women who have been depersonalised by the removal of their own clothes, who are all wearing a hospital gown either because it will prevent their own clothes from getting messy or because they have had an epidural, occupy rooms that all look the same—so similar-looking women are cared for in rooms which also look similar. Clearly, individual differences are being unravelled by hospital procedures and designs. The lack of individuality is no doubt particularly emphasised for doctors in the current system as they tend to go from room to room dealing with problems. They have less time to spend getting to know the women—unlike midwives who may, hopefully (given staffing levels), be in a position to form a relationship. Yet the women constitute a 'matching set' in which the individual components have virtually nothing in common apart from the fact that the women are all pregnant. One survey of one month's activity on a labour ward in an inner London teaching hospital revealed that only 34% of women were actually in labour, and so only 34% of the elements of the 'matching set' were in the process of giving birth or 'delivering.'

Exploring the use of the word 'suite' further, while the musical definition of 'suite' may seem totally unrelated, it is worth noting that the musical definition appertains to keeping something in 'order'. It is also worth noting that a 'suite of computer programs' is sold as a single unit, because all the programs in a suite are designed to work together. On a positive note, these last two definitions associated with the word 'suite' could be seen to reflect the wider multidisciplinary team work required for high quality care for women and babies during childbirth.

Despite the last positive interpretation of clinical teamworking, overall I feel the term 'delivery suite' has uncomfortable, middle-class and depersonalised connotations. The idea of matching sets and the emphasis on lack of individuality is inherent in the term 'suite'. Furthermore, when 'delivery' and 'suite' are put together, the message could be to subconsciously reinforce a depersonalised, mass-production approach of childbirth through the use of seemingly innocuous protective language.

Definitions of the word 'suite'

From: www.dictionary.cambridge.org/dictionary/british/suite_3:

suite *noun* (SET OF ROOMS)	a set of connected rooms, especially in a hotel
suite *noun* (SET OF FURNITURE)	a set of furniture for one room, of matching design and colour
suite *noun* (MUSIC)	a piece of music with several parts, usually all in the same key
suite noun (BATHROOM)	the set of fixed objects in a bathroom which includes a bath and/or shower, a toilet and a sink

From: www.dictionary.reference.com/browse/suite:

1. A number of things forming a series or set.

2. A connected series of rooms to be used together: *a hotel suite.*

3. A set of furniture, esp. a set comprising the basic furniture necessary for one room: *a bedroom suite.*

4. A company of followers or attendants; a train or retinue.

5a. *Music.* An ordered series of instrumental dances, in the same or related keys, commonly preceded by a prelude.

5b. An ordered series of instrumental movements of any character.

6. *Computers* . a group of software programs sold as a unit and usually designed to work together

When we use formal but quaintly depersonalised language we are guilty of hiding the raw awe and power of birth. We are also deceiving women about the immense challenge labour and birth poses for them and the potential for lifelong empowerment from it. Childbirth sits as a key rite of passage to full womanhood for many women and in many societies—but our terminology hides this fact. The 'delivery suite' terminology is like saccharine... it conjures up an expectation of middle-class relaxation, somewhat like a spa, but the reality is that it leaves a bitter aftertaste of the lived experience, which is usually a very clinically and medically orientated event in an extremely clinical and medical environment.

THE IMPORTANCE OF INDIVIDUALISED CARE

We must strive to deliver high quality individualised care to all women wherever they choose to have their baby. We do also have to have efficient and effective care for women and babies but while the model of the centralised labour ward may be the most efficient and effective use of clinical expertise I would like to argue that it is important to be aware of the subliminal pitfalls of the delivery suite' 'matching set' connotations.

In the next chapter I shall consider the emotional context for birth.

Exercises

1. This exercise will help you to explore what images words conjure up in your powerful subconscious. It is a valuable exercise to do either alone or with someone else. Take a pencil and five different pieces of A4 paper. Set a timer for a maximum of five minutes for each of the following words and draw images of the word. It doesn't matter whether you can draw or not—it is not quality and accuracy of the drawing that is important. What is important is that you don't use any words or letters within the drawing and you must draw pictures for the following words in the order given here: labour, ward, delivery, suite, motherhood. Now get up and do something else for a while and return to your drawings a little later.

2. Return to your drawings from Exercise 1. Can you see the subliminal messages you are sending to yourself from the pictorial portrayal of each word? If possible, show your drawings to a partner who has also undertaken the same exercise and see how your drawings differ from those of your partner. (An alternative to this exercise, which you could also try, or follow up with, is to play a version of the children's game 'Pictionary' where you try and get your partner to guess what you are drawing.)

3. Now think about three other words of your own choice, which are frequently associated with maternity care and repeat the drawing exercise, drawing three pictures in turn.

4. Think of five alternative names, either positive or negative, to describe the places women give birth in. What is it about words that makes them positive rather than negative?

5. Form a 'language guard', i.e. choose several colleagues or fellow students with whom you can work (as a small support group). It's helpful if you're all like-minded because your aim will be to help each other watch your use of language. Meet with one or two friends and challenge yourselves to see if you can eliminate language with negative or controlling elements from your vocabulary. Keep a diary and ask other people you are working with to point out when you are using words which you have all decided may be negative.

Further reading

Donnison J, 1988. *Midwives and Medical Men*. London: Historical Publications Ltd (2nd revised ed).

Downe S, 2004. *Normal Childbirth: Evidence and Debate*. Churchill Livingstone.

References

Care Quality Commission, 2010. Care Quality Commission Maternity Survey. December. Website: www.cqc.org.uk.

Donnison J, 1988. *Midwives and Medical Men*. London: Historical Publications Ltd (2nd revised ed).

Gould D, 2000. Normal Labour: A Concept Analysis. *Journal of Advanced Nursing, Vol 31, Issue 2*, pages 418-427.

Healthcare Commission, 2008. *Towards Better Births: a review of maternity services in England*. Commission for Healthcare Audit and Inspection.

Kitzinger S, 1992. *Birth and Violence against women: generating hypotheses from women's accounts of unhappiness after childbirth*. In Women's Health Matters Roberts H (ed). Routledge.

National Institute for Health and Clinical Excellence, 2004. Caesarean Section Guideline. London: NICE. Website: www.nice.org.uk.

National Institute for Health and Clinical Excellence, 2007. Intrapartum Care Guideline. London: NICE. Website: www.nice.org.uk/nicemedia/live/118737/36275/26375.pdf

Oakley A, 1993. *Essays on Women, Medicine and Health*. Part 1 The limits of professional imagination, p. 19-30, Medicine and Health, Part 1. and Consumerism and perinatal health, pp 52-63. Edinburgh University Press.

Royal College of Anaesthetists, Royal College of Midwives, Royal college of Obstetricians and Gynaecologists, Royal College of Paediatricians and Child Health, 2007. Safer Childbirth Minimum Standards for the Organisation and Delivery of Care in Labour. London: RCOG Press. Website: www.rcog.org.uk/files/rcog-corp/uploaded-files/WPRSaferChildbirthReport2007.pdf

Thornton T, 1998. *Wittgenstein On Language and Thought. Philosophy of Content*. Edinburgh University Press.

7: Ritualised care in the light of the evidence

*"As irrigators lead water where they want,
as archers make their arrows straight,
as carpenters carve wood, the wise shape their minds."*

Siddhārtha Buddha (circa 563 BCE to 483 BCE),
ascetic and spiritual teacher, and founder of Buddhism

IMPRINTING

Now that we have explored some of the backdrop of the power and politics being played out in maternity services, this chapter returns to the importance of setting the emotional context of maternity care. It also draws on comparisons from the animal kingdom to illustrate how important the first few hours of birth are to mother and baby.

Humans, like it or not, are emotional beings. And whether or not emotions are unruly, they are always powerful. They can overwhelm us, often when we least expect it, however rational and controlled we like to think we are. The ability to be hijacked by an emotion prevails throughout a person's lifetime. Emotions also are in essence timeless, in that through an emotional connection age fades into insignificance and the original emotional impact is still felt as a response throughout mind and body. These raw powerful emotions are often triggered by factors linked to early childhood experiences.

At exactly what point these trigger factors register on our unconscious is still under debate. We do know that learning starts *in utero*. Skin sensitivity starts to develop at about 8 weeks gestation. Taste develops around 14 weeks gestation and the sense of smell develops around the same time. It is believed that babies use these sensory experiences to understand smell and taste preferences in the mothers' diet and that these help babies identify and relate to their mothers when they are born. Reactive listening is functional from about 16 weeks gestation.

Although noise is muffled by amniotic fluid and other maternal body sounds, including maternal heartbeat, human fetuses are particularly responsive to voices and music.

The maternal voice is particularly powerful, probably because it resonates internally through the mother, as well as externally. A recent study has demonstrated that human fetuses not only remember sounds but also the melody and intonation of their mothers' voices. The newborn baby's cries then match the rhythm of his or her mother's voice, which makes both mother and baby both ready to initiate their relationship (Mampe et al, 2009). Given that this learning is taking place in utero, it is highly likely that the human mind also starts reacting and recording other events deep in its memory banks, while still in utero. This sensory information helps establish an early profound emotional connection between mother and baby which is going to be important for the baby's physical survival and to both mother and baby's longer term, emotional well-being.

It is not feasible to alter a great deal in utero although some women do play their babies classical music with a view to making their baby more intelligent. Even in circumstances where the mother is not going to be the primary carer for social or medical reasons, getting the baby to establish a strong emotional connection at the earliest opportunity with another adult is essential to his or her emotional well-being and in terms of developing the ability to relate to other people later in life. Once again this demonstrates that birth is not the end of a process, but rather a beginning. Therefore, it is essential to take every opportunity to build emotional resilience so that the baby is ready for the later challenges that life might bring.

In many animals, immediately after birth the newborn is hormonally primed for learning and imprinting, so that the baby can use its innate instincts to maximise survival (see 'Further reading'). For example, baby ducklings, as they hatch, fixate on the first object they see and then follow that object. Konrad Lorenz, a zoologist, reported on a now famous experiment where this happened when he hatched gosling eggs. One set of eggs were in an incubator and the other were with the mother goose. The goslings who hatched in the incubator saw Lorenz first and followed him, and continued to follow him even when later brought to the mother.

In many animals, immediately after birth the newborn is hormonally primed for learning and imprinting

Similarly, a baby wildebeest must get up and follow its mother, otherwise it is likely to be left to die. Baby wildebeests born during the migration season find themselves in large walking herds. In fact, pregnant female wildebeests congregate together to ensure that newborn wildebeests are protected from predators. If a pregnant wildebeest feels threatened during labour, her labour stops, and this can happen many times over. The only time labour does not stop is once gravity takes hold and the wildebeest's head and shoulders have already emerged. After they are born, since wildebeests migrate, the newborn wildebeest must get up and follow the first object they see, their mother, as their very survival depends on it—and baby wildebeests can walk within minutes. Female wildebeests are innately primed to reject baby wildebeests that are not theirs so the ability of the baby wildebeest to recognise and bond with its own mother is crucial and the first successful suckle at the mother's breast helps in this process through the sense of smell and taste.

Baby hippos are also interesting in this respect. They can walk, run and swim within minutes of birth. The mother hippo quickly teaches her baby to walk close by her side, usually level with her neck, stopping when she stops, so that she can watch the baby closely and protect him from aggressive male hippos. It is interesting that the greatest threat to a baby hippopotamus' survival comes not from other predatory animals but from other hippos.

Human babies are also vulnerable and totally dependent

Perhaps comparisons can be drawn with human babies as, arguably, they are so vulnerable and absolutely dependent on other humans for survival, being unable to even sit up, let alone walk, for many months. Human babies are dependent for much longer than other animals on adult carers. A human baby's dependency on the bond with his mother and father for physical survival is somewhat less obvious in our society, as others would feed and look after him if the parents didn't. However, like animals, human babies can also recognise their mother's voice and identify their own mother's breastmilk by smell. In a non-medicalised birth, our babies are also geared for survival by being so alert—they are wide-eyed, eager to make eye contact and mimic facial gestures, and able to attach themselves to the breast to feed. They are born keen to establish a good relationship with their future long-term carers, particularly their mother (Righard, 1992; Colson et al, 2008).

7: Ritualised care in the light of the evidence 79

Suspend your own personal belief system for a moment now and just consider the possibility that the treatment a woman receives during her labour and birth will be imprinting on her baby. Consider also that we are now caring for women in labour whose mothers and perhaps their mothers before them had increasingly medicalised births. The sounds of the labour room will be heard and possibly imprinted on the fetus, namely the voices, the mother's emotional reactions, the fetal heart-rate monitor recording their own heart rate in labour. This imprinting can happen in two possible ways: directly, through fetal sensory reactions to the sounds heard and chemical reactions in the mother's body at the time; and later, by word-of-mouth through mother to child, adolescent and adult discussions. For labour and childbirth experiences are one aspect of life that is almost always passed through the generations. It is also worth noting that women can vividly recall their experiences during childbirth throughout their lifetime. When women are dissatisfied with their birth, it is usually associated with the memory of the pain of labour and this plays a significant role in their longer-term memory. Positive experiences tend to remain interpreted the same, while negative experiences, particularly those which are linked to pain, tend to become even more negative over time (Waldenstrom and Shytt, 2009).

Already, in maternity services, we are increasingly seeing women expressing a lack of confidence in their ability to give birth without a caesarean section. It may take many more generations to manifest all the changes occurring in this cycle of life, just as it has taken many years to recognise the cumulative and longer-term problems associated with caesarean section, such as infertility problems, increased stillbirth rates and higher rates of life-threatening maternal haemorrhage and hysterectomy associated with placenta praevia and accreta (Solheim et al, 2011, Silver, 2010).

Are we, as humans, in our attempt to maximise immediate physical safety, missing an important element of care, i.e. that which involves facilitating the imprinting seen in other animals? Some believe it is our focus on immediate safety and our tendency to practise defensively because of increased litigation (for example, using fetal monitoring even though it has been shown to be of limited use) that are driving more obstetricians to resort to caesarean sections (O'Brien, 2005). It may be that when women and doctors are confronting having to have a series of hourly fetal blood samplings due to borderline results, and all the anxiety that accompanies these interventions, that they both, understandably, opt for what seems the safest option at the time. But although these immediate actions may ensure initial physical survival of some of our newborns, inadvertently, they may be having long-term deleterious effects on overall physical and emotional well-being.

Antenatal care, and in this I include antenatal education, was established with the purpose of improving birth outcomes and, according to Grantly Dick-Read, of ridding women of the dread of giving birth [1933]. Yet some would argue that our current antenatal care is only increasing women's fears. Many women come into antenatal care terrified of labour, with some requesting an elective caesarean section. So where does this fear originate? Perhaps this is another example of the presentation of imprinting during their own mother's labour and their experiences immediately following the birth. It could also be as a result of the influence and exposure of the media, which I shall discuss further in Chapter 9.

THE 'JUST IN CASE' MENTALITY OF MEDICALISATION

Generation after generation of women in the some countries of the world have now had the benefits of industrialisation, mass manufacturing and production of copious goods at relatively little cost. Innovation and technology have bought us easy access to intravenous infusion and safer operative outcomes. The pharmaceutical field has given us analgesic and anaesthetic drugs, antibiotics and artificial oxytocin. Advances in electronics have delivered us continuous fetal heart-rate monitoring and fetal blood gas analysis. All of these advances have insidiously permeated healthcare (Odent, 2002) to the extent that rather than being used to 'treat' problems, they have all at some time been used 'just in case' there is a problem.

The reason, of course, is that as our scientific knowledge has grown, we have started to consider our healthcare to be better than nature, even in the absence of complications. In Dublin this was made very explicit when the protocols involved routine amniotomy and intravenous infusion of syntocinon so as to ensure all women have their babies in 12 hours (O'Driscoll et al, 1984). Around the UK, and indeed around the world (eventually, if not immediately), continuous electronic fetal monitoring was introduced for all women in the 1970s without any evidence to support it. This started to be robustly challenged once the NICE published their fetal monitoring in labour guidance in 2001, and reiterated it in 2007. However, despite strong evidence to suggest it is unhelpful, continuous electronic fetal heart-rate monitoring (EFM) of low-risk women in labour is still prevalent in many maternity hospitals in the UK. Many midwives who have practised in this changing paradigm are still struggling with the changing concept of risk now associated with continuous monitoring. Having been told, for decades, since the late 1970s, that the risk to the fetus lay in not using continuous fetal monitoring, this procedure has been imprinted on their professional psyches. It is difficult for them to accept, 30 years later, that there is an increased risk to the woman with continuous fetal monitoring, i.e. the iatrogenic harm of an unnecessary caesarean section with all the associated complications. This changing emphasis on risk for fetal heart-rate monitoring is a manifestation of the law of unintended consequences which I alluded to earlier.

It is difficult for many caregivers, after decades of hearing the opposite, to accept the increased risk which EFM brings

Another illustration of unintended consequences was presented by Professor Greene recently at the RCOG Advanced Labour Ward Practice Course in March 2011. As he pointed out, electronic fetal monitoring can trigger feelings of both anxiety and reassurance in carers, women and birth partners. When all is going well, the fetal heart rate can be reassuring but if concerns arise, feelings of anxiety can creep in, escalating to fear and feeling out of control. Professor Greene shows film-clip evidence of midwives' and doctors' practices in birth rooms. In one of the vignettes, a woman who had had a previous stillborn baby is left alone in labour on a fetal heart-rate monitor and is seen to be trying to interpret the heart rate for herself. Professor Greene makes the point that these electronic fetal heart-rate 'monitors', as we call them, are only recorders of information and it is the doctor or midwife that is the 'monitor'.

Despite many technical advances, the ways in which a baby can be born have remained fairly constant, these being:

- ♥ spontaneously
- ♥ assisted with ventouse or forceps
- ♥ via surgical entry abdominally, otherwise known as a caesarean section

Sharon Oates, a consultant in obstetrics and gynaecology at the Royal Shrewsbury Hospital stated that a caesarean section is similar to having a 'hysterectomy', in an article in the Observer 2002. In medical terms, the suffix 'ectomy' refers to the surgical removal or cutting out (from Greek, 'ek' meaning 'out' and 'tome' meaning cutting). Commonly known 'ectomies' include tonsillectomy (the removal of the tonsils) and appendicectomy (the removal of the appendix). It is interesting that the surgical removal of a baby is not called a 'fetusectomy', which is technically correct, a 'babyectomy' or even 'a manual removal of a fetus under anaesthesia'. By giving the operation a name which has none of the traditional connotations with extensive abdominal surgery, it means we almost make a caesarean seem a more attractive option than a labour which is inevitably dominated by emotional and physical doubt and uncertainty—particularly if it is an elective caesarean section, which can be booked on a specific day to fit in with everyone's busy lives. Like other processes associated with birth, the caesarean section is seen as an end in itself and not the beginning of life, accompanied by recovery from the major abdominal surgery it involves.

Interestingly, the use of fetal blood sampling in labour, which can reduce the rate of unnecessary caesarean section, remains under-utilised. The reasons for this are far from clear. It may feel safer and easier to make the decision to do a caesarean section than await labour in the presence of concerns over a fetal heart-rate trace, given litigation and the consequences of making a mistake. For some reason, fetal blood sampling does not seem to be able to reassure clinicians sufficiently to give them the confidence in practice. They therefore opt for a caesarean section just in case. There is also the added complexity of the instant gratification which performing a caesarean section brings for the healthcare professionals. Once a caesarean section is performed, their job is done and if a healthy baby is born, all is well; there is in that 'moment' an instant feeling of relief and success. Furthermore, the act of performing surgery is itself attractive and rewarding to some doctors, as this is what they have been trained to do, i.e. it is their chosen career. The long-term ramifications of such a decision does not easily permeate a busy labour ward, dealing with life and death in the here and now. Fortunately, though, we are beginning to see greater scrutiny of the decision-making behind the high caesarean section rates today.

We are beginning to see greater scrutiny of the decision-making behind the high caesarean section rates today

DEVALUING THE POTENTIAL FOR EMPOWERMENT

The ventouse is a suction cup which is attached to the baby's head. It enables the skilled operator to aid descent of the baby by pulling, while the mother is encouraged to 'push'. In 1998 I once saw a doctor sensitively use the ventouse to aid descent of the baby down through the birth canal to the point of crowning (just about to be born), and then he deliberately detached the ventouse cup, enabling the woman to give birth to her baby herself, spontaneously . In this case, although the ventouse was necessary, only exactly the right amount of ventouse was used, so this was an assisted birth, not an assisted delivery. In other words, the doctor did not take control of the whole of the birth. This happened to be particularly important for this woman who I was caring for at the time and had a profound positive impact on her birth experience (Gould ,1998).

Despite this possibility of behaving in this way, this practice of earlier removal of the ventouse cup, at crowning instead of when the head is born, has never become mainstream. (Of course, if the ventouse cap should happen to come off accidently at this late stage, the doctors do always encourage the woman to push the baby out herself.) Why this practice has not become mainstream is pure speculation... It could be that it is felt to be too risky because the baby might not come after the cap is removed, possibly because it was taken off too soon. It could be that judging the time to remove the cap is too difficult. Or it could be that changing small things like this is not perceived to be an important aspect of care because it makes things just that little bit more complicated, and its potential for empowering the woman goes unrecognised. Whatever the reason, this is an example of how we sometimes seem to have difficulty refining medicalisation so as to really promote a sense of empowerment that some women can experience in childbirth. Instead, we allow our interventions to take over, rather than use just enough intervention to assist or facilitate the process. However, if we remove the ventouse cap earlier, there is a chance this might mean maximising the potential for those women (who need some help birthing their babies) to experience empowerment, and also minimising their potential for disappointment. The technique of using the ventouse cap with early removal is not meant to be used simply to shorten the second stage in otherwise normal labours, but it may well be appropriate for women who really do need an instrumental birth. Given the high epidural rate and associated need for instrumental birth, I think it is a great sadness that this idea has not been better embraced for those women who need assistance.

The potential for empowering the woman goes unrecognised

Early in my midwifery career women would, at 'transition' between first and second stage of labour—when labour is often at its height and women need to draw upon all their resources to get through—frequently be heard saying they wanted to' give up' and they would start asking for their mother, or plead that they wanted to go home. Presumably this is because these are both safe refuges for them, in a way. Today the pleas have changed and are much more medicalised. Today women tend to ask for an epidural instead.

Nurturing women through transition is one of the key midwifery skills which has been undermined by a culture which endorses an analgesic rather than a coping attitude to pain in labour. After all, if we meet those requests for an epidural as transition occurs, women are suddenly exposed to the epidural bundle of interventions, involving intravenous infusions, in-dwelling urinary catheter, syntocinon infusion, and instrumental birth. While many women will still be happy with this choice, for some women this decision will later be accompanied by a sense of disappointment in themselves.

The seismic shift which has occurred in recent years—from 'I want to go home' to 'I want an epidural'—will not be easy to undo. Any discussion about pain relief in labour is always inevitably emotive. It involves a real-life, almost daily clinical dilemma for many midwives working in hospitals where there is a 24-hour epidural service on request. They wrestle with the question as to whether it is their role to attempt to nurture women through transition or to go with the woman's request for an epidural, knowing as they do what it is likely to entail. The only way out of this and other potential clinical dilemmas is for the midwife to know the woman relatively well and for her to understand what is important to this woman during her childbirth experience. In a fragmented care model, this is unlikely, and the epidural will usually appear to be the safest option for all concerned. The result is a cascade of medicalisation and increasing associated interventions (and costs), although it must be remembered that refusing an epidural to a woman who really wants one can end up damaging her psychologically, which is also too high a price to pay. Therefore, if a midwife misjudges the moment of transition, when a woman calls out to her for help, she is also likely to feel guilty about the effect the decision made might have on the woman and she may also have to respond to a potential complaint as a result. And so the clinical dilemma continues, each one of us almost unwittingly playing a part in the medicalisation of childbirth.

RITUALISATION

Given the highly emotionally charged area of life that midwives and doctors work in, it is clear that problems may occur if caregivers start to feel stressed and unable to cope. There is evidence that healthcare workers may use ritual and stereotyping subconsciously to depersonalise women, so that they can emotionally protect themselves from the daily impact of dealing with life or death circumstances (Symonds and Hunt, 1994). Often these behaviours are subconscious and, when challenged, are considered seemingly irrelevant. It is therefore not surprising that small changes in behaviours are difficult to achieve, but it is disappointing if these small changes are not made, which cost little or nothing, given that they can have far greater ramifications than many people anticipate and given the improvement in care they can involve for women and babies.

Even today, following difficult births such as caesarean section or use of forceps, some newborn babies are placed out of reach and sometimes out of sight of their mothers at birth. This is often not done with intention to harm but the clinicians may still be caring for the woman, finishing their procedures, such as checking the perineum, suturing or preventing haemorrhage or other complications. This is precious time that is lost for all women but it is double jeopardy for women and babies who needed an operative birth because these are the very women who need to have the most intimate early contact with their newborn babies on account of the potential negative impact a difficult birth can have.

The Healthcare Commission Survey (2007), then later the Care Quality Commission (2010), curiously asked all women whether they had been sutured within 20 minutes of birth. The 20-minute timeframe rapidly became a target and marker of quality care. However, it is a marker that is not reflective of a sensitive individualised model of care which nurtures the mother-baby relationship from the start and, more importantly, it is not one which is based on any science—although I acknowledge that if a tear is bleeding significantly, in the interests of safety, it is wise to suture early. The 20-minute timeframe for suturing is the genesis of yet another but more modern ritual, designed to keep women from waiting many hours for suturing, but with unintended impact. In most cases suturing can be postponed so that early mother-baby contact is not disturbed.

It is not ideal for the woman's first contact with her baby to be interrupted by perineal suturing (unless the mother prefers for suturing to be done straight away), because of the immense importance of maternal-infant skin-to-skin contact immediately after the birth. It is incredulous that 20 minutes for suturing has become a quality marker when the practicalities of it might actually undermine quality care from an emotional and psychological perspective of welcoming the baby. After all, perineal suturing usually involves a vaginal and rectal examination and it is often undertaken in the lithotomy position. In the absence of an epidural, until the local anaesthetic is injected into the perineal skin and muscles, the woman will still feel pain as the local anaesthetic is administered and also during suturing if the local anaesthetic is insufficient during the whole of suturing. (If suturing is postponed, on the other hand, she will not experience pain during this 20-minute period.) Therefore, conditions are not ideal for mother-baby contact if suturing takes place within this 20-minute timeframe.

FEELING FOR THE NUCHAL CORD

During waterbirth midwives do not feel for a cord as they are practising the hands-off technique. Yet many midwives still feel for the presence of the cord around the baby's neck once the baby's head is born, when the baby is born in the air (out of the water). This has always puzzled me for if something is not a problem in water why is it a problem in the air? The procedure for feeling for a cord is not always without harm, especially if it results in early cord clamping or worse still, the cord snapping. The procedure can be uncomfortable for women, it can negatively interrupt the moment of birth and it may also cause labial lacerations, if done too energetically. If the cord is found, the three options are: firstly, to leave it alone and unravel it once the baby is born; secondly to try and pull it over the baby's head; and lastly, to clamp and cut the cord and unravel it.

If we are going to do nothing, as in Option 1, why do we feel for the cord in the first place? Option 1 is likely to have developed as a way of making the actual birth of the baby easier, so that the baby avoids being tangled in the cord at birth.

Option 2 involves potentially exposing the baby to a risk of cord rupture or snapping, and associated harm from sudden and sometimes significant fetal blood loss, if the cord is a tight fit over the baby's head. Furthermore, even after the cord is released from around the baby's neck, it is unlikely to increase the blood supply through the cord at this late stage.

The last option, which is still practised by some midwives, is perhaps one of the more worrying rituals. Once the cord is clamped and cut, the baby's blood supply is cut off. If there is then a subsequent shoulder dystocia, the baby will be without a blood supply. This could compound any harm that might come from shoulder dystocia and from the delay in the baby's birth. Even if the cord is tight, there is possibly going to be some blood supply, however small. It is exceedingly rare for a tight cord to be the cause of a baby not being born, it is much more likely to be because of a shoulder dystocia; so the practice of cutting the cord prior to the baby being born should only be done if the anterior shoulder is visible and if that is the case, there will be no need to cut the cord because the baby is about to be born anyway. Because of the risk of oxygen deprivation, the practice of clamping and cutting the cord before the baby's body is born should be used with extreme caution, and preferably not at all.

Given this discussion, it is surprising that the ritual of feeling for the cord is still a technique that is in practice. It may just be the fact that it makes the midwife feel that she is 'doing something'. Alternatively, it could be that knowledge has moved on from practice. In the presence of a tight cord, there is a technique described by Mercer et al (2001) where the midwife is encouraged to gently bring the baby up towards the mother, allowing him or her to somersault out and 'unravel' from the cord at the moment of birth (Mercer et al, 2001). It is worth remembering, though, that babies born in water do this for themselves.

FATHERS CUTTING THE CORD

Asking fathers if they wish to cut the umbilical cord seems to be another ritual introduced in an attempt to include them in the birth process. Many men take up the offer of cutting the umbilical cord. At the appropriate moment, the midwife dutifully hands over the 'special' cord scissors for the father to make the cut. This seemingly harmless way of involving fathers symbolically accentuates the baby's separation from the mother. It is much less common in our society for a woman to be asked if she wishes to cut her newborn's cord herself, even though other mammals separate their own babies by chewing the cord themselves. While for some fathers the ritual of cutting the cord has become a very important and symbolic moment of birth, there is little evidence that it promotes attachment. Instead, it may perhaps, somewhat controversially, create other subliminal messages of masculine power over women and childbirth

SKIN-TO-SKIN CONTACT

There is copious evidence on the benefits of maternal-infant skin-to-skin contact in terms of thermo regulation, regulation of the heart rate, increased breastfeeding success, and consequent easier adaptation to life. To date, there are no known negative effects of skin-to-skin contact between mother and baby at birth (Moore et al, 2007).

For many years, some highly medicalised maternity units have successfully managed to introduce skin-to-skin contact after caesarean section. They wish to promote skin-to-skin contact because they are aware of its known benefits. What is interesting is that in one of these units the person that pioneered skin-to-skin contact was not a midwife or an obstetrician, but an anaesthetist. This was an anaesthetist who had herself had an elective caesarean sections for her own babies. She had been supported by an obstetrician who had also chosen to have her babies born by elective caesarean section. Initially, it was the midwives who were negative towards the idea of skin-to-skin contact. However, the anaesthetist argued that fewer drugs were needed for pain relief when there was skin-to-skin contact and that women were more relaxed and happy following the birth of their baby when they could see and hold them close. (This is in addition to the benefits of skin-to-skin contact for the baby discussed earlier.) As a result, in the unit where those women worked skin-to-skin contact at caesarean section thrived. However in another unit, less than five miles away, skin-to-skin contact at caesarean section did not become the norm even five years later. Clearly, there is a vast difference in practices that cannot be accounted for by evidence or training. Skin-to-skin contact at caesarean section had become ritualised at the first maternity unit whereas the separation of woman and her baby was ritualised at the other unit.

In most maternity units around the country (and, indeed, around the world) women having caesarean sections are watching rituals being undertaken on their babies while they are powerless to join in. They are having their abdomen sutured while their baby is being weighed, checked, labelled and sometimes even dressed. If they are fortunate, their baby will be placed near them on completion of the suturing, but this is not always the case. Some babies' first few moments of life in this world are spent away from their mothers under the radiant heater of the resuscitaire to keep them warm. Why is that? It is partly because some obstetric theatres are kept at a temperature which is comfortable for the staff, and not for greeting a wet newborn baby—who needs a warmer environment.

There are still wide variations between units in skin-to-skin contact between mothers and babies. From this we can deduce that, somehow, it is likely that midwives are associated with either promoting or reducing skin-to-skin contact. I have heard many reasons given for this by midwives, including cultural preferences and the statement that women do not want to have the 'messy' baby skin-to-skin. I suggest if this is how skin-to-skin contact is promoted then probably they are right. Women would prefer 'dried and wrapped' because by the very language used we are suggesting that 'dried' implies wet and messy and 'wrapped' has links with gifts and a sense of being precious or prepared. Thus, the very language we use is influencing how women choose. The cultural argument is also not valid because the ethnicity of the women having caesarean sections was exactly the same as the women on the labour ward. How come, when on the operating table, women wanted skin-to-skin in the hospitals that provided it, but when they were supposedly in control they declined it?

Leading on from the debate about skin-to-skin contact at normal birth, it is interesting to note that increasingly there is also debate about whether or not newborn babies respond better to resuscitation when they are in close proximity to their mothers with the umbilical cord still intact, particularly if their mothers can touch their baby and are encouraged to talk to them (Mercer and Skovgaard, 2004). Of course, this is not how resuscitation is carried out in modern maternity hospitals. Usually, a baby's cord is immediately clamped and cut, and the baby is dried and wrapped and taken to a resuscitaire. This means taking the baby to a place where there is a radiant heater, light, a flat surface and equipment necessary to give lung-inflation breaths and, later, ventilatory breaths, if necessary, with equipment for intubation, should that be required. Whether or not a newborn baby would respond better to resuscitation nearer his or her mother is a very difficult issue, but we need to take into account the fact that the baby has already built a relationship with his or her mother and that he or she responds positively to her voice in utero. Mother and baby are also beginning to embark on their relationship in the outside physical world together so it would make sense for them to stay together at this key time. We know that people who are unconscious in an intensive treatment unit can hear and that they respond very positively when their loved ones talked to them... but we do not seem to easily translate this into practice around the moment of birth. Why would it be any different for babies? Is it not likely that talking to them might comfort them and help them respond? Is it that difficult to believe that a warm and loving mother might be attractive to her baby and that welcoming the baby into the world in her presence might make a difference? Why is it that when babies are sick, they are usually quickly isolated from their mothers? Once they are placed on resuscitaires or plastic boxes (incubators), there is often little if any maternal contact, and they are sometimes not even in sight of each other. (Of course, here, I am not talking about babies that need advanced resuscitation as this has to be slowly developed so as to ensure safety.)

How often have you been with an inexperienced paediatrician who is learning his or her job? Fearful of getting it 'wrong' and making a 'mistake', these inexperienced paediatricians are usually overly interventionist and reluctant to pass babies back to women. If a baby is relatively stable, it makes perfect sense to put the baby in skin-to-skin contact with his or her mother while the paediatrician watches the baby... but this is not undertaken very often because control would also pass to the woman. However, watching the baby in this fashion would require that new skills of observation be developed involving carefully watching while sitting beside the mother and baby. Perhaps by being so close, the doctor might feel overly vulnerable emotionally, because if inexperienced, this would be a scary time for him or her. It may be that just as we are increasingly expecting experienced obstetricians to work alongside inexperienced obstetricians on even routine calls, we might also need to require an experienced paediatrician to provide sensitive support in this kind of case, when a baby is just at the beginning of his or her life.

WEIGHING THE BABY

Computers and computer-related bureaucracy have become the tail that wags the dog in some maternity units. It is sometimes difficult to see how this can be altered in our current, increasingly rule-bound and compliance-driven culture. Babies are born and they are immediatly generated an NHS number. In order to generate an NHS number, the baby has to be computerised. The computerised data necessary for audit and data control require a baby weight. The baby is therefore taken from his or her mother and examined and weighed in the baby scales, often within an hour of birth. Some people argue that there is no harm in this as many women want to know how much their baby weighs. But is this not in itself another indication of how the rational scientific model has permeated society? After all, in healthy term newborns weight is irrelevant and in other cultures babies are not necessarily weighed. Weight becomes important only when drugs need to be given to sick or premature babies. Therefore, this is another example of the 'just in case' culture of 'only normal in retrospect'.

In normal circumstances, where is the sense of wonder at the baby being born? Why does the rational scientific model cut in so quickly? One reason, as I've pointed out, is because you cannot complete the computer programme without the baby weight. This anomaly has arisen because when the first computer programs were generated, healthcare professionals (probably midwives) said it was important to have the baby's weight because they were functioning in the 'throughput of work' model which involves tracking results. Now our information technology is driving the same rituals, and further embedding them in practice.

It is not only hospitals that drive this model. I was once told by one community midwife that it should only take one hour from the moment a baby is born to the woman and baby being fully processed, including baby being bathed, dressed, fed and the woman showered and transferred to a postnatal area. Today, there are still some 'work' teams that use this process model. As soon as the baby is born 'helpers' come in and start checking, labelling and weighing the newborn. The baby is fully dressed before the woman has had an opportunity to do anything.

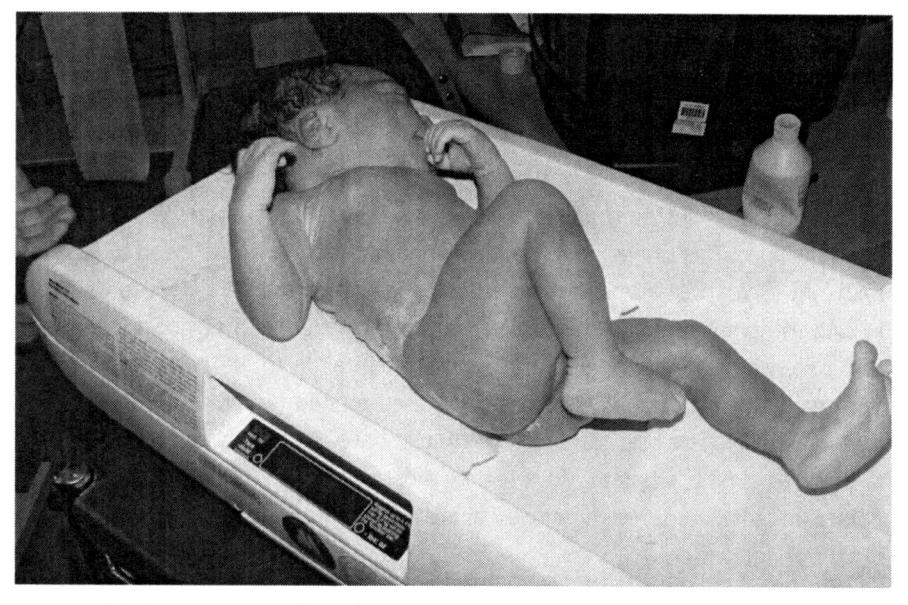

A baby—unnecessarily and prematurely isolated from his or her mother?

A NEW MODEL OF CARE

I have only chosen a few examples of ritualised care following the birth of a baby but there are many more. The important thing is to be aware of the role of ritualisation. It is easy to understand why we, as healthcare professionals, are exerting an influence over the mother's decisions: we are simply operating under the sick model of care, yet we are imposing institutional dominance over women in our care. However, the authority which comes with the status of being a midwife could be used to make a great positive difference to women and babies. In fact, it is surprising that it is not great technical advances which will make these differences to women and their families. It is small, seemingly unimportant actions which will make the difference and effect a shift in midwifery practice. This new practice will see these new, humane acts as normal. It will recognise that these changes which involve keeping the mother-baby dyad at the epicentre of care serve to promote and retain as much normality as possible, while still respecting safety as paramount.

This new model of care will involve imparting information in such a way that women will want to choose more normalising options. For instance, if you tell women that by having immediate skin-to-skin contact they will be helping their baby's heartbeat to stabilise, their breathing to establish and that it will keep them warm and therefore also protect them and help them adjust to life, I am sure that most women will willingly choose this option and do anything they can to help make it happen. I say this because of the lengths that women willingly go to antenatally to 'help' their baby. For some women, this includes painful invasive screening and several scans and blood tests. It makes no sense that any rational thinking person will stop wanting to do what is best for their baby the moment he or she is born. This brings us to another uncomfortable truth we need to face as midwives... We must admit that we are guiding women to make choices which fit in with the organisation within which we work, or even with our own biases. In doing so, we are tinkering with the natural adaptation to life process. Findings from my study into women's transition to motherhood (see Chapter 8) suggest that the small rituals associated with birth can have a powerful impact on women at this crucial time, when they are feeling most vulnerable and protective of their babies. In other words, our small rituals are important to women.

> Our small rituals are important to women. We must admit that we are guiding women to make choices which fit within the organisation within which we work.

For a moment just imagine that you are a fetus listening to your own heartbeat being monitored continuously, sometimes for hours during your journey into the world: a loud rhythmic pounding. Imagine hearing the midwives or doctors shouting "Push!" and "Push harder!" to your mother. It could sound frightening to someone listening, especially a helpless being listening from a darkened room. Imagine then being thrust into the world, struggling to breathe for the first time, only to be greeted by a resuscitaire or a cold set of scales, instead of being welcomed into your mother's warm arms and breast. What sort of imprinting are our current practices having on the female babies who will be childbearers in the future or on the male babies who may become fathers? The problem is that we may never know if any effects are fact or fantasy. Imagine for a moment that imprinting has been established for humans as a *fact* and these events act as key triggers for later emotional responses. Would the subliminal messages communicated by practices around the time of a baby's birth trigger positive feelings of self-esteem, love and caring, or self-hatred, anger and isolation? Would our childbirth practices be enhancing our society or destroying it? What would you change, given the chance?

The next chapter uses some direct experiences from women to explore aspects of how care might be improved to enhance maternal confidence and self-esteem following birth.

Exercises

1 Write down one sentence which best defines emotional resilience for you.

2 Take a moment to daydream. Consider if we are subject to imprinting at birth in the simplistic way that goslings are. If we are, who would the baby human first see in our labour wards and choose to follow? Consider this question for each of the following types of birth:

 ♥ a home birth

 ♥ a normal hospital normal birth

 ♥ an instrumental birth in a hospital

 ♥ a caesarean section

3 Write down the interventions that could help ensure that our human babies maximise their positive potential for imprinting soon after birth. What would you do differently or what would be different in the environment?

4 Reflect for a moment on why you think 'cutting the cord' has become so popular among partners. Consider what other actions do you or could you encourage fathers or partners to carry out in addition to the 'cutting of the cord' to help their relationship with their newborn flourish, without inhibiting the relationship between the mother and baby.

5 Write down one thing that you intend to do differently yourself using positive language. For instance: "I will positively promote skin-to-skin contact between women and babies." Place this statement in a prominent place where you will read it every day until it has become a habit.

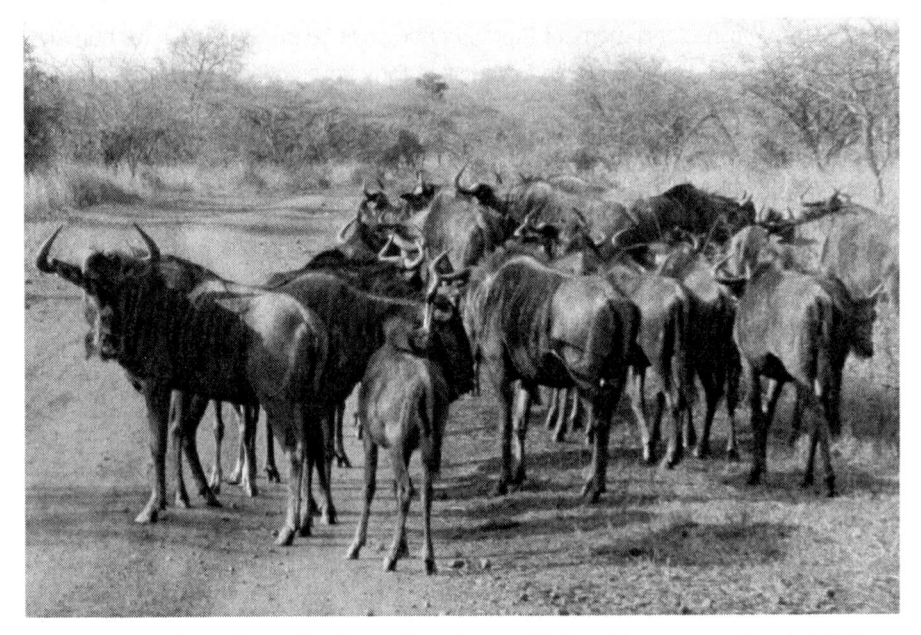

Considering how other animals—such as these wildebeest here—are primed at birth, how can we best make use of human babies' natural tendencies for survival?

Further reading

Hill A, 2002. Caesareans linked to risk of infertility. *The Observer*. Sunday 21 April.

Lonrenz K. Website: www.encyclopedia.com/topic/Konrad_Lorenz.aspx

National Institute for Health and Clinical Excellence, 2001: Electronic Fetal Monitoring: The use and interpretation of cardiotocography in intrapartum fetal surveillance. London: NICE.

National Institute for Health and Clinical Excellence, 2007. Intrapartum Care Guideline : management and delivery of care to women in labour. London: NICE.

References

Care Quality Commission, 2010. Maternity services 2010. Website: www.cqc.org.uk/aboutcqc/howwedoit/involvingpeoplewhouseservices/patientsurveys/maternityservices.cfm

Colson SD, Meek J, Hawdon JM, 2008. Optimal positions for the release of primitive neonatal reflexes stimulating breastfeeding. *Early Human Development*, Vol 84, no 7, July, pp 441-449.

Dick-Read G, 1933. Childbirth Without Fear. Heinemann Medical Books. (Reprinted by Pinter & Martin in 2009.)

Gould D, 1998. Assisted birth not assisted delivery. *Midwifery Matters*. September, p 3.

Healthcare Commission, 2007. *Women's experiences of maternity care in the NHS in England. Key findings from a survey of NHS trusts carried out in 2007*. London: Commission for Healthcare Audit and Inspection.

Mampe B, Friederici AD, Christophe A, Wermke K, 2009. Newborns' cry melody is shaped by their native language. *Current Biology*. Dec 15;19(23):1994-7. Epub Nov 5.

Mercer J, Skovgaard R, 2004. Fetal to neonatal transition: first do no harm. In *Normal Childbirth: Evidence and Debate*. Soo Downe (ed). London: Churchill Livingstone.

Mercer JS, Skovgaard RL, Peareara-Eaves J, et al, 2001. Nuchal cord management and nurse-midwifery practice. *Journal of Midwifery and Women's Health* 50(5):373-379.

Moore ER, Anderson GC, Bergman N, 2007. Early skin-to-skin contact for mothers and their healthy newborn infants. Cochrane Database of Systematic Reviews, Issue 3. Art. No: CD003519. DOI: 10.1002/14651858.CD003519.pub2.

O'Brien P, 2005. Stemming the rising caesarean section rate. *British Journal of Midwifery*, 13(5):328.

Odent M, 2002. *The Farmer and the Obstetrician*. Free Association Books.

O' Driscoll K, Foley M, MacDonald D, 1984. Active management of labor as an alternative to cesarean section for dystocia *Obstetrics and Gynaecology*, April, Volume 63, Issue 14 p 485 -490

Righard L, 1992. Delivery Self Attachment. Video. California: Geddes Productions.

Silver RM, 2010. Delivery after previous cesarean: long-term maternal outcomes. *Semin Perinatol*. Aug;34(4):258-66.

Solheim KN, Esakoff TF, Little SE, Cheng YW, Sparks TN, Caughey AB, 2011. The effect of cesarean delivery rates on the future incidence of placenta previa, placenta accreta, and maternal mortality. *J Matern Fetal Neonatal Med*. Mar 7.

Symonds A and Hunt SC, 1994. *The Social Meaning of Midwifery* Palgrave Macmillan.

Waldenstrom U; Schytt E, 2009. A longitudinal study of women's memory of labour pain--from 2 months to 5 years after the birth. BJOG: *An International Journal of Obstetrics and Gynaecology*, 116(4):577-583.

8: Facilitating the transition to motherhood

"The mother-child relationship is paradoxical and, in a sense, tragic. It requires the most intense love on the mother's side, yet this very love must help the child grow away from the mother, and become fully independent."

Erich Fromm (1900-1980), German-American Jewish social psychologist, psychoanalyst and philosopher

THE CINDERELLA SERVICE

Following discussions in the last chapter on the importance of the first few hours following birth in the animal kingdom and possible effects on the mother-baby relationship in humans, I shall now use the experiences of women as a canvas to illustrate where we can look to improve the care we give to women and babies in our hospitals following birth. Postnatal care has long been considered the 'Cinderella' of maternity services, i.e. unloved, overworked and neglected. As long ago as 1987, Ball carried out extensive research into 'reactions to motherhood' which led her to describe birth as 'a peak life experience in the life of parents, a deeply emotional and personal moment which cannot be recaptured' (Ball, 1987, p. 137). She asserted then that emotional needs are often neglected at this time due to the task-orientated approach to care. This lack of attention to emotional support for women and their families in the postnatal period is still prevalent today, as demonstrated by the Healthcare Commission Review into Maternity Services (2008), the Care Quality Commission (CQC) Survey into Maternity Services (2010) and The National Childbirth Trust Survey (2010).

Motherhood... "a peak life experience... a deeply emotional personal moment, which cannot be recaptured"

The National Childbirth Trust Survey (October, 2010), aptly named 'Left to your own devices', surveyed the postnatal care experiences of 1,260 first-time mothers. 42% of women who responded said they had not received all the emotional support they needed in the first 24 hours following birth, with a third of all women saying they received little or no emotional support in the first month after birth. Nearly half of the women did not feel they had been given all the information and advice they needed about their babies' health, and over half of the women said they had not received all the information they needed with regard to their own health and well-being.

This was echoed by the CQC Survey (December, 2010) which found that approximately a fifth of women felt they did not get enough information about their own health and recovery following childbirth and that they were unprepared for the emotional aspects of becoming a new mother.

UNDERSTANDING WOMEN'S FEELINGS

In order to better understand the feelings, emotions and perceptions of women in the first few hours of motherhood I carried out a research project into women's experiences of the transition to motherhood and presented my findings at the International Confederation of Midwives Conference in Vienna in 2001. As not much seems to have changed in women's experiences of postnatal care in many of our hospitals, given the findings from these recent surveys, I thought it relevant to share these findings now. Doing so may shed some light on areas to focus efforts in order to improve care for women following childbirth.

The study took a phenomenological approach, which means trying to understand the 'lived experience' from the perspective of those experiencing the event. The question I was interested in was 'What are the feelings, emotions and perceptions of women in the first few hours of motherhood?' By asking an open question, I was able to look afresh at women's experience of the first few hours of motherhood from the sole perspective of the new mothers. I wanted to discover the 'essence' of this experience by exploring it through the pre-reflective descriptions of those who had very recently lived it. The women chosen were a purposive sample of women having their first baby, who had had a normal birth at term, and had English as their first language.

I used a semi-structured questionnaire to keep focused on the first few hours of motherhood, using a topic guide I constructed from a literature review and from my personal experience as a midwife. First of all, I asked the women in the sample: "In your own time and words, can you tell me everything you can remember about your feelings, emotions and perceptions around the time your baby was born?" I then used the following trigger words as a topic guide during our interviews:

- first seeing baby
- atmosphere
- feeding
- events after the birth
- people present

My research involved interviewing five women for approximately an hour each. (All the women freely consented and their anonymity was guaranteed, so their names have been changed on the following pages. The relevant ethics committee approval was also obtained at the time.) Although a small-sample phenomenology relies on richness and depth of data from in-depth interviews, I acknowledge that the small sample size is a limitation of the findings to some extent. The interviews were taped and then transcribed by myself so I could immerse myself in the data to enhance my understanding. All of the women had given birth within 12 to 24 hours of the interviews taking place. To ensure the validity of my findings, so that I could be confident that what I found reflected what the women had said, I sent them a copy of their typed-up, taped interview for them to verify for accuracy and also involved them in verifying the categories and findings—and they made no changes. At the point of categorising the content of the interviews into themes, I involved another midwife researcher so as to get an independent view of accuracy. (This procedure, which is called using an 'interater', also improves the validity of findings.)

Shock or surprise

All of the women I interviewed expressed some degree of shock at the impact that labour had had on them. They all reported a memory of intense pain during their labour. They also described feelings of either shock or surprise around the time of the actual birth of their baby. For some, this sense of shock brought on feelings of emotional numbness, which they had not expected, and this shocked them further. For others, although there was a sense of relief that labour was all over, it was accompanied by feelings of embarrassment about some of their behaviour while they'd been in the throes of the pain of labour.

All of the women recalled feeling frightened in labour. For example, one woman said: "The room was just like we'd been left in an operating theatre (laughter) and you did wonder what was going to happen next". (Claire) This feeling was accompanied by feelings of loss of control, of feeling unable to cope, with one woman stating that she had 'given up hope'. (Annie). Other women commented as follows:

♥ "When I thought he started to be delivered I thought 'I can't cope with this.' You know, I can't. I just got hysterical." (Becky)

♥ "My prominent thoughts and feelings are about the last 20 minutes when he was coming out. It was so painful. That's the most outstanding... it's that and him being put on me... After going on for hours and hours, suddenly for it to pop out like that I thought 'Wow, great.'" (Claire)

♥ "My labour shocked me. It is a shock to the body. I was shocked at the birth and I am really shocked about my feelings (for the baby). Perhaps I feel a bit numb (crying)." (Evelyn)

And one woman described her sense of embarrassment following labour:

♥ "When it doesn't hurt you think 'Oh my God... What a fool I have made of myself now.'" (Claire)

These feelings of shock and embarrassment pervade early motherhood and for some women can arouse feelings of low self-esteem and emotional numbness, which increases their vulnerability just when they need to feel strong and confident in their role as a new mother.

The women in this sample were relatively well following the birth of their baby, having had an uncomplicated birth. The NCT Survey (2010) found that the early postnatal experience was worse for women who had had operative births. These women reported even greater dissatisfaction with their care, support and the information they were given about their own and their baby's health. 43% of women who had had a caesarean section felt that little or none of their emotional needs had been met in the first 24 hours following birth. In addition to these feelings, if they are typical, women who have had a caesarean are likely to be experiencing more physical pain or greater incapacity through intravenous infusions, urinary catheters, or epidural analgesia wearing off. They are also more likely to have experienced and be recovering from postpartum haemorrhage as defined by a blood loss of more than 500 ml. As a result, these women are likely to be more vulnerable and more in need of support than the ones I interviewed for the research project.

THE NEED FOR EMOTIONAL SUPPORT

What became apparent through these interviews is that midwifery behaviours have a direct impact on how women feel. This can have a powerful positive influence on how women deal with and overcome their immediate sense of vulnerability after they have given birth.

All of the women interviewed described their need for support. They were very grateful for sensitive midwifery support, especially if it helped them retain or regain a sense of control. Some of the women talked about midwives who positively supported them more like friends. These particular women all had partners with them during labour and they also gave substantial recognition to the support their partners had given them in labour.

The way partners are treated in the early postnatal period is also important. Many hospitals ask partners to leave once the woman is transferred to the postnatal ward, if their baby has been born at night. When their partner has left, the new mother is often left alone with her new baby, hence the title of the NCT survey report into postnatal care being called 'Left to your own devices' (2010). This behaviour suddenly isolates the partner after going through the intensely emotional experience of seeing his (or her) baby born. Yet the early postnatal period is a crucial time when partners could provide more support by helping new mothers with their baby while they rest a little… or they help even if they just spend time with the mother, so that those first few precious hours with the new baby are experienced as a family. In the NCT Survey (2010) women said they would have felt less vulnerable and 'scared' if their partners could have stayed with them overnight. Some hospitals are beginning to extend visiting to enable partners to stay longer but the lack of availability of single rooms for immediate postnatal care does seem to inhibit this initiative at night for most women and their partners.

ADAPTATION TO MOTHERHOOD

The intensity of the emotional support women acknowledged and appreciated from their partners during labour and birth seemed to bring the couple together. However, almost as soon as their baby was born, these women reported that the dynamics in the relationship with their partners subtly changed. Although this change was to some degree expected because the women had known they were going to become mothers, it also exacerbated their feelings of uncertainty. One woman described the sudden profound change in relationship dynamics that her first baby had brought, simply lamenting: "It's such a change from two to three." (Annie)

> "It's such a change from two to three."

Adaptation to motherhood in this early stage has many facets and the new status takes time to sink in. Common themes identified that could be categorised under adaptation to motherhood include responses to thinking they would fall in love at first sight, and their emotional reaction when this did not happen as they expected.

One woman described how she felt: "I thought I'd be really happy because I've got Down's syndrome and spina bifida in my family. I've already had lots of tests and things. He is so perfect. Why can't I love him like I thought I would?" (Evelyn)

Another described how their baby did not really feel like it was theirs, and how she felt she still had not moved on from pregnancy: "While I was feeding her it was as if I could still feel her moving inside me, as if I was feeding someone else's baby. I thought that was quite funny considering she was right in front of me." (Annie)

Yet another woman told how she felt the need to hold her baby close in an effort to get to know him but felt somehow guilty doing so. She had not yet internalised that this was her baby and that she was in control of her mothering style. "I keep picking him up. I know I shouldn't but I want to." (Danielle)

Some of these feelings may be generated by the proliferation of baby books giving very different perspectives on mothering, including Gina Ford's sometimes contentious *Contented Baby Book* (Vermillion, 2006) which focuses on the presumed importance of establishing routines.

THE IMPORTANCE OF TELLING FAMILY & FRIENDS

All the women described how they wanted to tell family and friends about their newborn baby as soon as possible after the birth. Friends and family seem to be extremely important in validating the new reality for women following childbirth. This early contact with family and friends carries a sense of immediacy about it and serves to consolidate the woman's new status as a mother. If this does not occur soon after birth when women want it to happen, there can be feelings of limbo generated which prolong a feeling of unreality, as if the rite of passage has not quite been completed. One woman summed this up when she said: "I haven't seen anybody yet so it's all a bit of a dream at the moment." (Danielle)

Another woman said: "I want to go home, he doesn't feel like he belongs to me at the moment." (Claire)

Clearly, for some women there is a period of time when their own baby feels slightly alien to them. Friends and family seem to have a strong role to play in integrating a woman's transition to full motherhood in their own society following birth. Proactively, establishing early links back into their own lives may be crucial to well-being and may aid maternal-infant attachment. In a society where many people are separated from the larger family, friends may play a more important role in consolidating the full status of the role of 'mother' on a woman, immediately after she has had a baby.

FEELINGS OF PROTECTIVENESS

Four out of the five of the women had strong protective feelings towards their baby. These women expressed great concern and anxiety if they were separated from their baby for any reason. In addition, the sudden heightened responsibility of motherhood weighed heavily on them. It was as if the protectiveness and responsibility for the baby's well-being intertwined. "All of a sudden there is this young baby here that is not going to go away. I don't feel this way about anything else. I've *got* to look after him." (Claire)

For some women, this overwhelming sense of responsibility drives them to want to do everything 'right'. This need for perfection in caring for their baby leads to a lack of confidence, as it is impossible to be perfect with a new baby. This is further compounded if conflicting advice is given, or if women receive a lack of support with their babycare routines, such as changing their baby's nappy, feeding or bathing. It is during this early adjustment that some women lament their lack of experience and knowledge of baby care and this can also undermine their confidence. "It is so scary. You are frightened you don't know what you are doing. You've got to hope that you do it right. (Tearful) Here we go... It's like labour." (Evelyn)

These women craved for simple non-contradictory practical help and information so that they could get things 'right' and establish some kind of control. Some women had prepared for this event by reading about baby care. However, they expressed disappointment that the literature didn't match their lived experience, which was far more fluid and less amenable to being prescriptive than they had anticipated.

For some, the feelings of responsibility were overwhelming and they searched for reinforcement of their ability to care for their baby, in order to allay their anxiety. When the feeling of protectiveness was strong and the responsibility of it felt overwhelming, the women seemed to lack confidence in themselves, and so were not able to relate well to their babies in the initial hours.

"I've got to learn what to do with this thing. It doesn't come automatically when you are pregnant. You need to be taken step by step through slowly. Now I am a mum I've got to sort it out so I mean to learn and be confident. Make sure I am doing it properly and then I will feel successful." (Evelyn)

It might be the need to establish control of an uncontrollable element, another small person, that drives some women to establish 'routines' early, so as to fit the baby into their lives. Alternatively, it could be that hospital rituals and routines over the course of pregnancy, childbirth and during early postnatal care give women the subliminal message about the need for ritual and routine at home. In this way, it is possible that our institutionalisation of maternity care may not only be medicalising childbirth but also creating dependence on rational scientific models for early infancy and mothering. As mentioned before, this is compounded by baby gurus who all seem to have the definitive parenting guide, when what women need to do is to be able to trust their own instincts.

It is possible we contribute to a perception that routines are needed

It seems that the early period following birth is a time of huge emotional turmoil, when tiredness, hormonal influences and feelings of emotional overload create potential for disappointment. One suprising finding of my study was that all the women stated that they appreciated an opportunity to talk about their unexpected feelings. This suggests that women feel vulnerable after childbirth, unsure of their status and in limbo between maidenhood and motherhood because they have experienced birth but not yet become fully-fledged mothers.

Primitive responses of protectiveness are triggered in some women and these can further increase their anxiety, if women feel unable to care for their baby or if they doubt their own ability to do so. In some women these feelings can rapidly spiral into worry and lack of self-esteem in the early postnatal period. The alien hospital environment also adds additional difficulties as women are trying to reconcile their primitive emotional responses to childbirth, including a sense of responsibility and protectiveness, with the physical and psychological stimuli of their hospital environment. All of the women in the study experienced feelings of guilt and anxiety when they were separated from their baby, even when they were still close. For example one woman explained: " I didn't like the fact that they have to take them away, but she did the measuring on the bed next to me, right next to me. It's a funny feeling because you know nothing is going to happen, he is right there and you can see him. It is just a peculiar feeling. You feel so protective. You don't want anyone near him." (Becky) Clearly, women are aware of the dangers of being separated from their baby in the hospital environment, particularly the risk of baby abduction.

One woman said: "I was very concerned about going out of the room and leaving her because of the Abbie Humphries case." This was a high-profile case of a baby who was daringly abducted from a Nottingham Hospital in 1994 by a woman dressed in a grey uniform, pretending to be a healthcare worker. The mother, who happened to be a midwife, had left to make a telephone call when the abductor, Julie Kelley, tricked the father into handing Abbie over to her to go for a hearing test and left the hospital. Abbie was not found for 17 days. Even if women are aware and concerned by this case, women still seem to accept a degree of separation in the hospital environment. "The only time I have been separated is when ... he went for a hearing test. I felt fine with that. These are people [midwives and staff] I've trusted." (Claire)

In this case the women trust the healthcare workers in hospital and use this to mitigate their feelings of protectiveness for their baby. Many units today have security tagging to alert staff if a baby is being removed without warning. Some also have automatic lockdown systems that lock the entrance doors when the alarm is triggered. Fewer hospitals are still choosing to use the presence of security guards positioned outside postnatal wards and at entrances to maternity units.

IMPLICATIONS FOR PRACTICE

A welcoming-baby model would honour the new mother as principal carer for her baby from birth. However, this does not mean abandoning her to provide care but it is a model which offers kind, sensitive support, which reinforces the mother's efforts and helps to build her fragile self-esteem and confidence. It involves creating a nurturing, virtually ritual-free zone, in which the new mother can better explore and deal with the inevitable ambiguity and uncertainty that becoming a mother brings. In other words, we need to start mothering new mothers in the most positive sense, nurturing their innate ability to care for their babies in their own way from the moment of birth onwards.

> A welcoming-baby model would honour the new mother as principal carer for her baby from birth

Routine separation of new mothers and their babies is thankfully unusual today. However, there may still be some times when a woman and her baby are separated and it is important that staff know how best to support women if this has to occur. In these cases every effort must continue to be made to keep women and their babies together, especially for routine activities like neonatal examinations and hearing tests.

Early discharge home for healthy mother and baby to expedite adjustment to motherhood is also important. Nevertheless, this must be supported by models of care in the hospital which reinforce the importance of family and friends, not by a model of care which sees them as a nuisance and which tries to exclude them from contributing in the early hours of motherhood. Early discharge also requires supportive models of care in the community setting.

> Early discharge, with support in the community, is also important

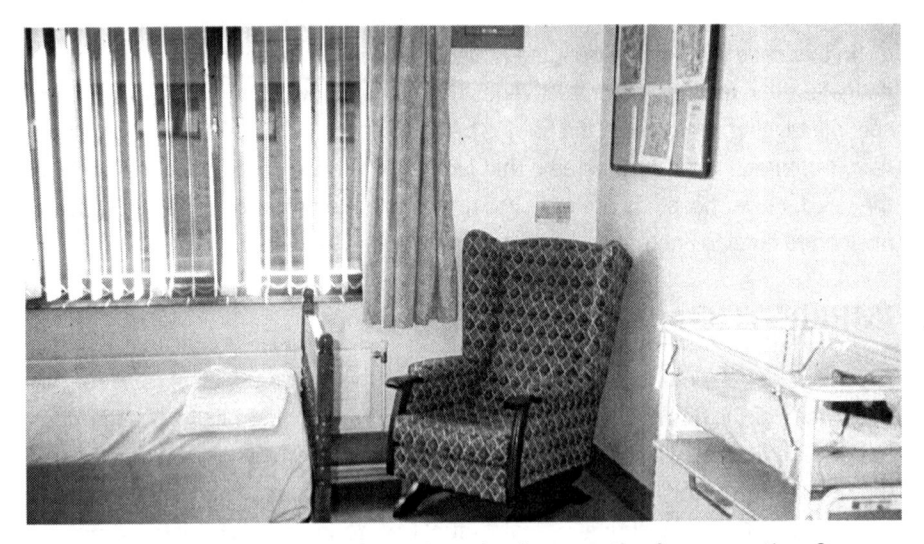

How can postnatal rooms be made optimally supportive for new mothers?

It is vital that we raise awareness of the 'rite of passage of birth' and develop strategies to reinforce every woman's transition to motherhood. After all, while labour will have unfrozen aspects of the woman's core identity, it is important that the highly vulnerable state of 'limbo' associated with the transition to motherhood be acknowledged by healthcare professionals and women and their families. By raising awareness of this transient state, we might be able to help women adjust more easily to motherhood and better understand how to help women minimise unnecessary increased anxiety. This could be done by listening, informing and supporting women's decision-making, while always encouraging their independence and boosting their confidence as mothers. Flippant comments can be particularly damaging at this stage as women in limbo, who are highly anxious, tend to receive information in a very literal manner. This is probably because during an opened emotional state such as 'limbo' during a rite of transition the subconscious can be directly accessed and there is no help from the conscious, critical faculties in the brain—so women are unable to criticise or reject information being received. All healthcare providers need to understand this in order to give positive empathetic support to women when they are in transition, on their way to motherhood. However, on the positive side, this vulnerable, open, psychological state also offers a window of opportunity to plant positive suggestions and build self-confidence in women's mothering abilities without the conscious mind rejecting this new confidence.

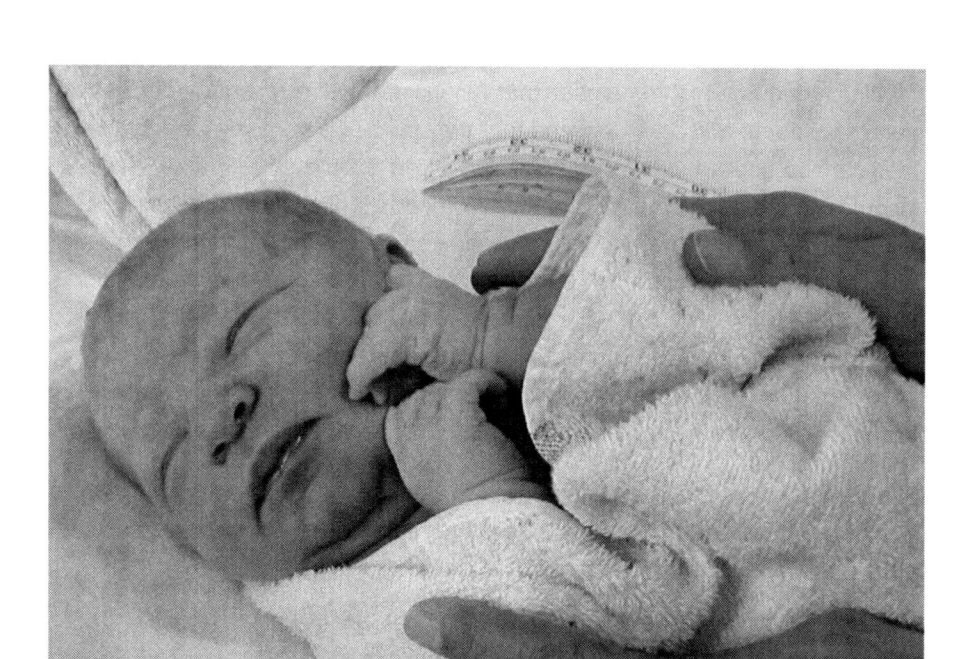

We need to remember the value of gentleness when dealing with newborn babies. After all, these little human beings really do seem to have feelings.

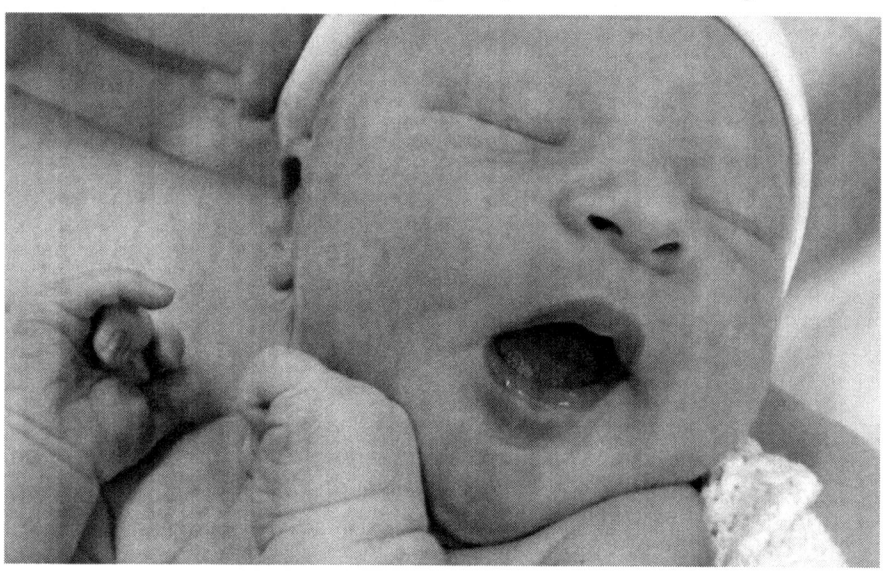

Finally, we need to remember that family and friends are a quintessential part of childbirth and parenting and that they provide a necessary link between medical and social models of care. Every effort should therefore be made to incorporate the involvement of family and friends, if the woman wishes this, in the early hours of motherhood. This may mean that in the future our hospitals have to change their approach and facilitate visiting by providing rooms during the night, if women do not have a single room, and facilitate visiting at other times by providing private rooms, rather than ward areas for visiting. Exploring how to safely enable partners to remain with women and new babies in hospital is of critical importance for all maternity service managers.

The importance of the interaction between women and their family and friends is widened in the next chapter as it discusses the mismatched perceptions of birth in the media and in real life.

Exercises

1. Divide a sheet of paper down the middle. On the left side write down words to describe five attributes you would ascribe to the character Cinderella in the well-known fairy tale. On the right hand side, using each word you have written on the left hand side describing one of the attributes, write a sentence about postnatal care. For instance, you might write the word 'poor' on one side to describe Cinderella and on the other side you could write. "Postnatal care has historically been under-resourced in comparison to the rest of maternity care so is often seen as a poor relation." Once you have done this for every attribute reflect on the metaphor of Cinderella for postnatal care and consider how valid you think this metaphor is in reality.

2. If childbirth is a rite of passage to motherhood (and full womanhood for some women) write down how well you think we are currently meeting women's needs, giving our performance a score out of 10, with 10 being the highest. If you feel we deserve a score which is less than 10 write down specific examples of where we could do better.

3. Are there some simple acts or behaviours that could positively impact on women's well-being that we are currently not doing? If so, can you commit to introducing just one intervention where you work so as to improve things yourself?

4 Think for a moment how we could reduce the anxiety associated with women's overwhelming feelings of needing to 'protect and look after their baby'. Write five sentences describing specific actions that, if carried out, could boost a woman's confidence. Now underline any verbs in the sentence to highlight the actions which need to be implemented.

5 What are the barriers to change? On a piece of paper mark down against the sentences above those things which are totally in your control and those that are not in your control. Commit to changing at least one that is in your control.

Can you commit to introducing just one intervention where you work so as to improve things yourself?

Further reading

Davis-Floyd R, 1993. Birth as an American Rite of Passage (Comparative Studies of Health Systems & Medical Care). University of California Press.

Mercer J, Skovgaard R, 2004. Fetal to neonatal transition: first do no harm. In *Normal Childbirth: Evidence and Debate*. Soo Downe (ed). Churchill Livingstone.

Murphy J, McMahan I (ed), 2006. The Power of Your Subconscious Mind: One of the Most Powerful Self-help Guides Ever Written. Pocket Books.

References

Ball JA, 1987. *Reactions to Motherhood*. Cambridge University Press.

Care Quality Commission, Dec 2010. *Care Quality Commission Survey into Maternity Services*. Website: www.cqc.org.uk/aboutcqc/howwedoit/involvingpeoplewhouseservices/patientsurveys/maternityservices.cfm

Ford G, 2006. *The New Contented Baby Book*. London: Vermillion.

Healthcare Commission, 2008. Towards better births, A review of maternity services in England. Commission for Healthcare Audit and Inspection. Website: www.cqc.org.uk

The National Childbirth Trust, Oct 2010. Left to your own devices: The postnatal care experiences of 1260 first-time mothers. Website: www.nct.org.uk

9: Mismatched perceptions in the media and real life

"Whoever controls the media, controls the mind."

Jim Morrison (1943-1971), lead singer and lyricist of the American band 'The Doors'

A MISREPRESENTED EVENT IN LIFE

The paradox of birth is that it is a uniquely extraordinary event, yet at the same time so commonplace as to be ordinary; this fact haunts its portrayal in the media. It really is a very common event, since over 700, 000 babies are born every year in England and Wales (Office for National Statistics (2010). This means that almost everyone, somewhere in their extended family, will be welcoming a new baby at some time during each year. Therefore, the extraordinary uniqueness of uncomplicated spontaneous birth is often lost in the media melée because it is so 'extraordinarily ordinary' that it is not news. In addition, despite the enormous number of babies being born every year, birth is usually a very private affair. Nevertheless, the way in which birth is reported in the media—which only reports on unusual or celebrity cases—could potentially have a profound influence on how women perceive the safety of childbirth.

We now are beginning to see a voyeuristic interest in birth creeping in with the advent of fly-on-the-wall TV documentary programmes such as *One Born Every Minute* (available to view at www.channel4.com). This programme films the experiences of women during pregnancy and childbirth, as well as the experience of midwives in a large maternity unit in the south-east of England and was shown on television in the UK during 2010. It can sometimes make uncomfortable viewing as it provides a glimpse of how the uniqueness of birth and the relationships that surround it can be tainted by the commonality of labour and birth that is the midwives' and other staff's daily experience—although the midwives on the whole have to be commended for the standard of care delivered in a very busy maternity unit. Programmes such as these reveal the reality of midwives' daily working lives... At times they show what a real difference midwives can make in the lives of women and their families, but at other times they also depict another angle altogether. I say this because although *One Born Every Minute* is ostensibly about birth, I have heard colleagues talking about the behaviour of the staff who appear on the programme, including the midwives, and not about the women or their families, or the birth itself.

Therefore, even when birth is laid open for all to see, the nuance of the life-giving moment is lost and instead people find themselves thinking about how people do (and should) behave around birth, and healthcare workers find themselves considering the normality of doing their job so candidly on camera. Clever editing has meant that glib comments, patronising statements, and everyday habits and behaviours from midwives and other staff occasionally cut the air, leaving splinters of the shattered illusion that midwives and other staff treat every woman and birth as special and unique. The close-up shot of the large staff teapot which appears repeatedly in the programme raises the interesting question as to whether the programme is about birth, midwifery or midwives, who are only human after all, with all the normal strengths and failings of any human beings. Many midwives I know cannot bear to watch the programmes but it was immensely popular with the viewing public and it slowly felt more like a soap opera or sit com, so made good TV. Therefore, even when the media's intention is to capture the powerful moments of birth, this still doesn't appear to be interesting enough without the candid shots of staff and tea, which turns life into satire and brings satire to life. Even the short promotion film emphasises this point with a conveyor belt of babies being shown to the tune of 'Whistle While You Work' from the Disney film *Snow White*.

In the media, much like war, pregnancy and birth are often portrayed as very boring most of the time but sudden crescendoes are also included which are anxious moments of intense life or death activity. However, in the case of birth, the romance and sexual tensions which often appear in war films are virtually never depicted. Instead, birth is portrayed as a sterile event, when it is filmed for popular media. Usually, birth happens on a bed in the middle of the room, with the woman lying or sitting in a semi-recumbent position. The constant movement of women in normal labour, with their rocking, swaying and walking is translated to rolling in distress from side to side on a bed. The deep guttural noises associated with normal birth, which have sexual connotations, are translated into screaming distress. Women are portrayed as passive participants in birth, have things done to them, rather than as active participants, as if they were weak, overcome and almost possessed by this entity called birth. In portraying birth in this way, the sexual nature of birth is avoided in the same manner as penetrative sex is banned from usual viewing on our TV screens. It is as if birth is portrayed in the old Hollywood movie fashion, where stars like Doris Day and Rock Hudson, when filming 'love' scenes in bed, had to keep one foot on the floor to ensure decency. The sight of a baby's head fully distending the vagina as it crowns is virtually never seen. Instead, the scene is cut or the shot reverts to the clock on the wall, as if the camera were seeking anything to ground us back in the 'real' world of material things, measured time and a sense of control. This filming approach operates just like some dark mysterious mirror which unconsciously reflects the very clinical rituals, discussed in earlier chapters, which currently surround birth in the developed world, with its emphasis on time and weight.

Our newspapers are no different. Most 'news' items dealing with birth are usually linked back to hospitals and clinical labour ward environments which are then eagerly photographed or filmed and used as a backdrop for the 'news', sometimes, for no other reason than the assumption that equipment like fetal heart rate monitors, ultrasound scanners, incubators and operating theatres make 'good' pictures that make 'good' stories, which is, after all, what the media are essentially about. One recent example of this was in *The Guardian*, on 1 January 2010. Cathy Warwick, General Secretary of the Royal College of Midwives, had published an article outlining her concerns about the lack of midwives and midwifery input into maternity care and the dangers associated with this. The large picture alongside the article did not depict midwifery or normal birth, but a naked newborn baby being held aloft by a woman in theatre scrubs wearing rubber gloves and the backdrop looked like an obstetric theatre.

CONSEQUENCES OF INACCURATE PORTRAYAL

When childbirth is depicted in our TV soaps and sitcoms, there is usually a lack of interest by writers and producers in the long, drawn out, repetitive contractions of the first stage of labour. As a result, in the media version of birth everything is speeded up. Labour often starts with a sense of urgency to get the woman to hospital from the very first contraction or her membranes rupturing. This urgency, as labour begins, is usually acted out with high anxiety and trepidation rather than with joyful anticipation. This combination of urgency and trepidation emphasises to the viewing public that birth is risky and underlines that hospital is the safest place for birth. It also encourages women to go to hospital as soon as they are in labour and conveys a message to partners that getting to the hospital early is the right thing to do and that part of their role is to ensure this happens. This is despite evidence that women in early labour are better off staying at home, where they can relax in their own environment and wait for labour to become established. Hospital admission in early labour is associated with increasing likelihood of unnecessary medical interventions, including caesarean section. It is also associated with emotional disappointment in women who are often advised that they are not yet in labour and that they need to go home to wait for labour to become established. Since the message from the media has penetrated so deeply, this can spark fear and anxiety in both the woman and her partner at a time when they need to be relaxed, calm and preparing for the labour to come. But once fear and anxiety set in, it is also very difficult for midwives to convince women that home really is the best place for them at this stage of labour and many insist on staying. For those women who cannot be persuaded to go home, some of them may then be inappropriately admitted. However, as the early stage of labour often lasts many hours and there is little to distract women in the hospital environment, women become despondent, they feel they have been in 'labour' for a very long time and then they start to think that something is wrong. This scenario sets off a cascade of spiralling interventions, often beginning with an epidural, moving on to syntocinon augmentation, continuous fetal heart rate monitoring, suspected fetal compromise and possibly forceps or ventouse, or even caesarean section.

> Once fear and anxiety set in, it is very difficult
> for midwives to convince women that home
> really is the best place for them early on in labour

When labour is portrayed as taking a long time, the underlying assumption is that there are life-threatening complications. I do believe that most writers and television and film producers want to make their stories realistic, but perhaps they have difficulty doing this because of the mundane normality and length of time labour can take, involving little overt activity, which conflicts with their need to stimulate and thrill an audience.

SUBLIMINAL MESSAGES ABOUT BIRTH

This medicalised focus and incomplete portrayal of the realities of birth give substantial subliminal messages to people not previously exposed to birth, for we must remember that the majority of people have no direct experience of birth itself, so they have no other reference point, other than what they see in the media. Subconsciously, the message is paternalistic, conveying that birth is inherently dangerous, and that early hospitalisation and copious medical equipment is essential. Sadly, the whole of our society has been indoctrinated with this message since the advent of television in everyone's home. It is entirely possible, although difficult to prove, that the portrayal of birth through television itself is partially responsible for the rising rates of interventions and caesarean section. After all, it is also through the media that different stakeholder groups try to get their message across and once again, just as publication bias affects research evidence, the interventions of obstetricians are more likely to provide 'good' viewing , whereas a midwife skilfully watching, waiting and supporting the moment of birth does not. Although some TV and filmmakers do try to depict the natural progression of labour in a positive way, the majority do not and, in failing to do so, they may be unwittingly leading women into an interventionist cul-de-sac which is almost impossible for midwives to get them to reverse out of. Since there is such a huge gap between the media messages being received into people's subconscious and their effects in real life, the associations and connections between the media and women's experiences of childbirth are difficult, if not impossible, to prove. The unenviable challenge for media professionals is how to be realistic and deliver a positive message to women while still providing a product which will be successful in terms of attracting viewers, plaudits and publicity.

So even before a woman becomes pregnant, the seeds of the baby-danger metaphors are already in place for many women and pattern-matching occurs rapidly. There is only a small window of opportunity from beginning of pregnancy to onset of labour to try and change that mindset through factual information giving. However, factual information giving will reside in the conscious mind and take a while to be accepted deep in the subconscious mind and, ultimately, it is the subconscious mind that really governs attitudes and behaviours in all of us. Meanwhile, even during this window of opportunity, the media are constantly reseeding people's brains with their powerful baby-danger metaphors which sterile, factual, antenatal education classes will do little to assuage. The baby-danger metaphors are indelibly printed on the psyche of the nation.

Once the woman comes into hospital, the baby-danger metaphors she is so familiar with through media coverage are instantly reinforced by what she sees in our traditional labour wards, whether she is conscious of this or not. This may be why some women report that they are reassured by medical equipment on show when they go into hospitals with highly clinically-orientated environments. This reaction is curiously illustrated by the playwright Nina Raine's award-winning reflection on her experience of shadowing doctors and nurses in hospital, which she did to research a new play. When hearing the interview, you get the distinct feeling that this artist and observer of humanity is more than a little uncomfortable disclosing her own reaction to the hospital environment when she describes how she found 'comfort' in the pristine clinical equipment. I suggest this gave her back a sense of control and safety in the overwhelming and uncertain world of hospital and disease. For example, at one point in the interview (published in The Metro, on 11 January 2010) she says, with a small laugh: "There's something very comforting about hospital paraphernalia. You get this diseased asymmetrical body ravaged by cancer and then these lovely clean syringes". (Allfree, 2011). Although her reflections are focused on ill health, her comment reveals how clinical equipment and, by implication, medical interventionist care, is perceived and portrayed as a metaphor for healing and 'comfort'.

Contrast this possibly unconscious view of labour and birth with the messages midwives are trying to give women when they become pregnant. We are trying to offer women a choice of place of birth from home to midwifery-led birth centres and labour wards, but if women who are the second or possibly even the third generation growing up exposed to medical media stories, which do you think they are most likely to choose? With 9 out of 10 partners being present during labour and birth, where do you think the partners will want their babies to be born?

The growing demand for epidural and the likely subsequent cascade of interventions could in part be because of the media's relentless focus on the 'dramatic and unusual'. Or it could be because of the common depiction of women screaming in pain, often with a focus on the second stage of labour, with the woman pushing and screaming. Worse still, it could be because the woman is portrayed as being insignificant, with the focus being on the partner.

The growing demand for epidural and the likely subsequent cascade of interventions could in part be because of the media's relentless focus on the 'dramatic and unusual'

REVEALING MEDIA STORMS

When one professor of midwifery, Denis Walsh, tried to widen the debate around labour, pain and the promotion of coping mechanisms to women giving birth in hospital, there was an immediate backlash in the media. Walsh advocated the use of yoga, hypnosis and immersion in water to promote normality, help reduce interventions associated with epidurals and he also dared to mention that in doing so, maternal-infant attachment might be enhanced. Headlines such as 'It's good for women to suffer the pain of a natural birth, says medical chief' (*The Observer*, 13 July 2010) led the attack, which was backed up by quotes from women from various networking websites which helped the media to polarise the issues. The debate became increasingly newsworthy since Denis was a male midwife: he was portrayed as a man who was telling women what to do in childbirth, something that as a man he would never have to experience himself. The emergent division between the sexes portrayed in the media and in online network sites was interestingly further exploited for public attention when a Radio 4 interview featured 'Denis, the male midwife' talking about these issues with a female obstetrician. The media rollercoaster ensured that emotions were shaken and stirred, and the rational message Denis was trying to convey, which many women support—which went against the prevailing medicalised view of childbirth—was largely ignored.

Monty Python's film *The Meaning of Life* has a depiction of birth in a maternity unit labour ward which satirises both the modern view of childbirth and the media portrayal of birth. This portrayal is unique in that the sketch highlights how modern technology and medical management have so overtaken the birth process that the woman is lost amongst it. At one point, when everybody is in an operating theatre literally full of equipment, John Cleese notices that something is missing—and that 'something' happens to be the woman herself. Before this, the focus had been on the new piece of equipment, the machine that infamously goes 'bing'. While this is funny, it is like all good satire in that it leaves the informed feeling desperately uncomfortable; it is a salutary reminder that childbirth can become depersonalised, without people even noticing that this is happening, when staff are exposed to it every day. To prevent depersonalisation I believe it is vitally important for midwives and doctors to ensure that a relationship is built with the pregnant or labouring woman, however small an amount of time there is to do that.

The opportunity to incorporate important health messages into soap opera storylines is what many medical professionals and the charities aligned to them often aspire to. However, the BBC1 soap EastEnders that was popular for 25 years and watched by more than 10 million viewers, saw its producers having to defend their New Year baby swop plot which prompted over 6,000 complaints from viewers. In the storyline over the New Year, one of the characters, Ronnie Branning, has a baby who suffers a cot death, and she secretly swaps her dead baby for another character's baby. Ann Diamond, a presenter who herself has campaigned for cot death awareness since losing her own son, accused the producers of trivialising the issues and going 'one step too far'. This outcry is a prime example of how certain truths are exaggerated or twisted to make reality even more 'dramatic' in the name of entertainment. John Yorke, the controller for BBC Drama Production, was interviewed about this storyline and he said that although the BBC conduct research to make their storylines real, he emphasised that "our job is to be a drama." The Cot Death Society (www.cotdeathsociety.co.uk) supported the use of cot death in the storyline but they also condemned the baby swap plot. The outcry and subsequent defence of this sad storyline is one of the clearest examples of how the media, particularly drama, manipulates events around childbirth so as to satisfy our craving for entertainment (BBC News, 6 January 2011).

> This is an good example of how the media manipulates events around birth so as to satisfy our craving for entertainment

INTERESTING GAPS IN MEDIA COVERAGE

It is curious to note that for a subject that holds endless fascination, pregnancy and birth do not figure highly in the emergent gaming industry. This is strange given that other sinister aspects of life, including war and rape, are explored and played out in the very realistic gaming industry involving adult games. For example, war is the background to *Call of Duty* and its sequel *The Dark Arts* and rape and death are included in a car-theft chase game called *Grand Theft Auto*. Given the EastEnders twisting of fate in its cot death storyline described above, on reflection perhaps it is actually a good thing pregnancy and childbirth have eluded such exposure. After all, it is difficult to imagine how a gaming industry which focuses on thrills and extremist, dramatic, action-packed experience would advance the cause of understanding the importance and power of birth.

A REALISTIC APPROACH TO THE NEWS

Midwives and other health professionals reading this should note carefully that birth is usually only interesting to the wider media when technology and machinery are involved, when the birth is unusual, when it contains a dramatic emergency, when it occurs in an unusual place, when it is attended by an unusual person or when it involves women screaming in agony. The (BAFTA British Association of Film and Television Awards) award clip makes this clear (see 'Suggested viewing' at the end of this chapter).

> Planned home birth is not news in the UK

Planned home birth is not news in the UK. However, a baby being born at home, unplanned, unattended or attended by a person other than a midwife or doctor means that the person present becomes a local hero and that is 'news'. Even a devastating 'cot death' is not 'dramatic' enough for some.

Maternity care stakeholders must also remember that the media's *primary* interest does not lie in portraying high quality evidence-based maternity services, however much we may lust to lure media magnates into promoting normality alongside us. Normality in all its stark glorifiable simplicity does not make, and is unlikely to ever make, good television, sell newspapers or become an online sensation.

Nevertheless, media attention, including film and television, can be a gift to midwives because it gives us an opportunity to criticise things from a distance, from a possible place of safety (e.g. in antenatal appointments) and explain some of our core cultural beliefs and behaviours so that we can see how other people see them. This is useful because, after all, raising awareness is always the first step in any change process.

> Media attention can be a gift to midwives because it gives us an opportunity to criticise things from a distance, from a possible place of safety and explain some of our core values

The next chapter takes our increased awareness of the influence that core values have on thinking and decision-making a step further. It suggests that we could learn from the spa experience so as to improve how we nurture women during childbirth.

9: Mismatched perceptions in the media and real life 119

Media reports presenting an unrealistic overview of birth

Twin baby girls share a single body

About a woman in China who gave birth to conjoined twin baby girls who shared a single body—appeared in *The Sun* in 10 May 2011

Giving birth in California more dangerous than Kuwait or Bosnia?

About the worrying tripling of mortality rates in California—appeared in the *(NY) Daily News* on 3 Feb 2010

Beyoncé and Jay-Z take an old-fashioned approach to pregnancy

About the celebrities, who were criticised for conceiving naturally, unlike other celebrities who had IVF and unusual relationships—appeared in *The Telegraph* on 31 August 2011

Cruz: Motherhood is 'beautiful'

About the celebrity Penelope Cruz, who says she changed 'immediately' after giving birth—appeared in *The Express* in 10 May 2011

Epidurals: time to stop labouring over 'natural' childbirth

About the apparent supremacy of epidurals since labour is compared to Olympian exertion—appeared in *The Times* in 27 March 2008

Obesity blamed as more mothers die in childbirth

About the rise in maternal mortality, which is attributed to increasing BMIs in mothers—appeared in *The Times* in 04 December 2007

Exercises

1. To help understand the raw emotional impact the media has on people and on childbirth itself, try this colourful exercise. Gather together a piece of paper and some coloured pens, pencils, or sticky paper. The more colours you use, the better!

    - Be quiet and think for a minute about a portrayal you have seen of pregnancy and or childbirth in fiction, media stories, on televisions or in a film. Make the image very vivid in your mind.
    - Now use the coloured pens, pencils or sticky paper to represent the emotions the image conjures up in you, not the detail itself. You can use as little or as much colour as you wish.
    - Take a break.
    - Now revisit the colours you have chosen. Do they represent balance and calm or fear and uncertainty, achievement or loss?
    - Finally, think what words you would now associate with your colours and write them on the same sheet of paper.

2. Take another sheet of paper and repeat the exercise above, this time thinking how you would like to see pregnancy and birth presented ideally. Use colours first, then add words afterwards, as you did before.

3. Now look at your drawings and writing from Exercises 1 and 2 above and compare and contrast what you did for Exercise 1 and 2, noting the key differences, if any.

4. Lastly on a scale of 1 to 10, with 10 being the highest, rate how much influence you think you or the midwifery profession currently has on the presentation of childbirth in the media. Score again to indicate how much control you think we might have in the future. Write down the five key reasons for scoring each of these at the level you did.

How much influence do you think we have on the media now?
How much influence might we have on the media in the future?

Further reading

Campbell D, 2009. 'It's good for women to suffer the pain of a natural birth', says medical chief, Derek Campbell, Health correspondent. *The Observer,* 12 July. Website: www.guardian.co.uk/lifeandstyle/2009/jul/12/pregnancy-pain-natural-birth-yoga (Accessed 5 June 2011).

Suggested viewing

Monty Python: The Meaning of Life—Available at www.dailymotion.com/video/x1sh3y_monty-python-the-meaning-of-life-bi_fun

One Born Every Minute: promotional video: baby production line—Available at www.dailymotion.com/video/xiderk_one-born-every-minute-promo_shortfilms

One Born Every Minute: clip from the series—Available at www.youtube.com/watch?v=nnW3VM-x7QY&feature=relmfu

One Born Every Minute: BAFTA award speech—Available at www.youtube.com/watch?v=TJms1iFnxMw&feature=related

One Born Every Minute, programme—Available at www.channel4.com/programmes/one-born-every-minute/episode-guide

References

Allfree C, 2011. Dedications in the detail Interview with Nina Raine. *The Metro,* January 11, pp 40-41. Website: www.Metro.co.uk

Office for National Statistics, 2010. Website: www.statistics.gov.uk

BBC News, 2011. EastEnders-Cot Death Baby Swap Storyline Complaints on BBC News. Soap archives, 6 January.

10: From conspiratorial models to an inspirational approach

"If you're remarkable, it's likely that some people won't like you. That's part of the definition of remarkable. Nobody gets unanimous praise—ever. The best the timid can do is be unnoticed. Criticism comes to those who stand out."

Seth Godin (1960-), American entrepreneur and author, from 'Purple Cow: Transform Your Business by Being Remarkable', page 45

BE REMARKABLE!

As I have said, the first step towards change is to raise awareness and first of all we need to do that within ourselves. If we are going to move from conspiratorial models of care to an inspirational approach, we are going to have to go deep inside ourselves first and deal with our own attitudes and beliefs on a deep psychological level. But beliefs are interesting and powerful... You cannot force someone to believe something. Once a deeply-held belief is established, even in the presence of concrete proof to the contrary, people may not necessarily change their mind about it. A good example of this is the long-held belief that the world was flat, long after it was proved that it was not.

Inner beliefs are often overlooked, yet they are so powerful they can either create or destroy lives, organisations and civilisations. The conscious mind only takes care of the small fraction of what is being processed. It is the subconscious mind with its bank of internal beliefs which is the hidden but major decision-maker. Messages are bombarding the body the whole time from all the five senses, sight, hearing, touch, smell and taste. The subconscious mind makes decisions all the time and often instantaneously. Therefore, in daily life, there is relatively little time to influence decision-making, because it is in a moment that people choose to do or not do something. It is in a moment that a midwife chooses to follow hospital protocols rather than adjust care to better suit the needs of that individual woman and her family. It is in the moment that ritualistic care is re-enacted rather than care which is carried out in a loving and meaningful way. There is substance to the saying that old habits die hard, because habits are built on established belief systems and they are reinforced by repetition. Sometimes, in our daily activities, decision-making is so fast that individuals who make the decisions are not even aware that they have made a decision at all. Furthermore, many people also need reminding that no decision is also a decision.

Given all of this, before we talk about how to move from conspiracy to inspiration, it is important to realise that seldom do we as midwives mean deliberate harm or offence to people entrusted in our care. We are actually responding in a way which maximises our personal sense of survival as our subconscious mind perceives it. This reaction will be based on our own inner-belief system, whether we are aware of it or not (Murphy, 2006). In addition we may not even be aware of the full impact of our unconscious thoughts on our behaviour. As adults, we will have deep-rooted belief systems which have been built up over time, with many having been laid down in childhood, spread across family, social and also work environments. These beliefs have become interwoven as a result of life events from infancy on, and they include the professionalism of training and the institutionalism of our workplace. It is these belief systems that need to be adjusted if we are really to move ourselves and everyone we work with to a position where we aspire to make the time around birth the best it can possibly be for both mother and baby, and also their wider family.

By re-engaging in what made you become a midwife, and getting your colleagues to do likewise, I believe you can help overcome the conforming-to-institutional behaviours, as revealed by Kirkham (2004). Kirkham's work showed that midwives often knew that the care they were delivering was not evidence-based or woman-centred but, unremarkably, it allowed them to live a more peaceful work life with colleagues.

As I explained in Chapter 4, many midwives find the aspirations which brought them into the field of midwifery originally are soon quashed by the daily reality of their working lives. What really perpetuates this gap between aspiration and reality? It is easy to blame lack of resources, resulting in understaffing, a lack of equipment and poor décor, but it goes deeper than this. I have worked in many hospitals in my career both in modern hospitals which are well-resourced and also in older, less well-resourced ones within the NHS and I have found that while resources are important, the provision of sensitive, quality maternity care is as much dependent on the values, attitudes and behaviours of the people delivering the service as on the resources themselves.

Beliefs are interesting and powerful.
You cannot force someone to believe something

In overly medicalised environments, resources can be squandered on unnecessary equipment and sometimes invasive tests which, rather than add to quality care, actually detract from it. Midwives and doctors can feel pressured and frightened by having to directly engage in the emotionally supercharged event of birth, the beginning of life, and perversely feel they are living in the shadows of death daily instead. The need to confront the extremes of life and death so regularly and so profoundly does not feature in any other aspect of health care. It is as if midwives are servants to the realms of life and death, slavishly trying to make the passage to life as easy as possible, yet all the while recognising that sometimes they have to soothe the suffering that death brings. This is all the more poignant for, as midwives, the majority of us concentrate on bringing in new life, although there are a few specialist posts specialising in bereavement. Our very nature ensures that we identify more strongly with life than death and the closer death encroaches, the more precious life becomes. This is especially the case with childbirth, where we witness not only the birth of a newborn baby but also the metamorphosis of a woman into a mother.

To really change how people behave and start to protect the time of birth, we need to break the cycle of individual dependency on group acceptance, to further reduce tolerance of medicalised norms and celebrate the moment of birth rather than greet it with professional sighs of relief. Therefore, training and education (which includes in-service training) need to focus first on who the carer is, what she or he values and why she or he has decided to come into maternity care. Much can be gleaned about what we value by exploring what drew us into the profession in the first place. Rarely is the reason that it is a reliable and well-paid job.

Midwifery nearly always attracts people who want to make a positive difference in the lives of others and who marvel at the uniqueness of childbirth. Midwives have also often been touched in some way by birth experiences in their early lives, a time when inner belief systems are being formed. This is a powerful force to harness because when you are trying to change behaviours, if you can tap into a long-held belief which makes up a 'core value', you will find that the conscious part of the individual will not dismiss the message you are trying to get across. Techniques from neuro-linguistic programming and hypnotherapy which encourage relaxation, positive suggestion and anchoring, can all be used. This can be either within groups or individually, to help create positive behaviours and group values which reinforce the sanctity of the woman and her family. The importance of pregnancy and childbirth can be amalgamated with the valuable aspects of medical knowledge and skills into a social, emotional and spiritual framework creating a new paradigm that will benefit everyone. This will help everyone receiving or delivering maternity care to be able to experience real 'meaning' in their lives and it will create an improved sense of well-being for all.

We need to release core values, attitudes and behaviours that drive midwives to advance advocacy and accountability with pride and determination, rather than retreat in passivity and be silently overwhelmed by institutional norms.

MOVING TOWARDS A MEANINGFUL MODEL

In order to move towards a model of midwifery which is more meaningful, as I've explained, it is vital that we re-engage with our core values regarding care for women, and that we help other midwives to do this too. How can we do this? Corporate standards and external compliance doctrines of minimal accepted attitudes and behaviours are unlikely to have a profound impact on deeply ingrained attitudes and behaviour so we must tap into personal motivation. Often core values have been suppressed by other competing personal and emotional needs for survival. Perhaps there is a fear of bullying, a need to be liked and accepted, a wish to avoid criticism and failure and even, for some, a wish to avoid too much success. As discussed in depth in Chapter 4, Deming (1992), in his total quality management model, states that fear and inspection are actually inhibitory of quality. He advocates that the best way to deliver quality is to inspire staff to want to deliver the highest standards for their own sense of pride and satisfaction, not to be compliant with a certain standard.

Once midwives are re-engaged with their own core values, the personal commitment to deliver high quality care will increasingly overcome institutional norms, especially if these values become embedded in the organisational culture so that work once becomes meaningful and is therefore no longer just 'work'.

The highlighting and reframing of individual and group core values will help to illustrate how some current working practices, such as unnecessary rituals and routines, and production-line maternity care, conflict with these belief systems.

This may provide the first crack in the mirror of current cultural norms which reflect back the rationale of the scientific model, professional hierarchies and organisational priorities which still underpin many modern maternity services. Once you and your colleagues have explored and re-ignited your core values deep in your subconscious, this should pave the way for infinite change and raise your own and your colleagues' consciousness, so that you more willingly reject previous attitudes and behaviours which conflict with your sense of work which brings meaning.

> Once you and your colleagues have explored and re-ignited your core values, this should pave the way for infinite change

One factor which I believe underpins the success of this model is our innate human striving for happiness—and this ultimately crosses all cultures. While human beings undoubtedly enjoy sensations of pleasure, it is the longer-lasting inner feelings of happiness that almost all people really want. Pleasure may provide an emotional high but its effect is short-lived. Whereas pleasure might be derived from a group, for example when colleagues tell you how well you are working, true happiness is more than that because it is not just about feeling good. As Hoggard points out (2005), happiness involves a sense of real commitment to living life well and being able to make value choices in life which generate an inner sense of meaning.

Value decisions are choices made that keep you aligned with core inner values which reinforce your individual and collective sense of meaningfulness. Delivering care from this basic model of meaningfulness will eventually become easier and easier because you will find that early initiatives generate a sense of inner happiness within yourself and your colleagues, which will then make you want to continue with a more caring paradigm. Anthony Robbins (2001), a guru in self-development, believes that it is in the single moment that a decision is made and destiny determined. He emphasises that it is the thinking about the decision that takes time. If this is true, it can only be by changing how we think in the lead-up time to the moment of decision-making that we can change the type of care we provide. It means it would be pointless trying to influence any decision as it is being made, as there is simply not enough time in that precise moment to effect deep enough change. Raising awareness of how we make decisions and how belief systems and ways of thinking affect the decisions we make, is the first step.

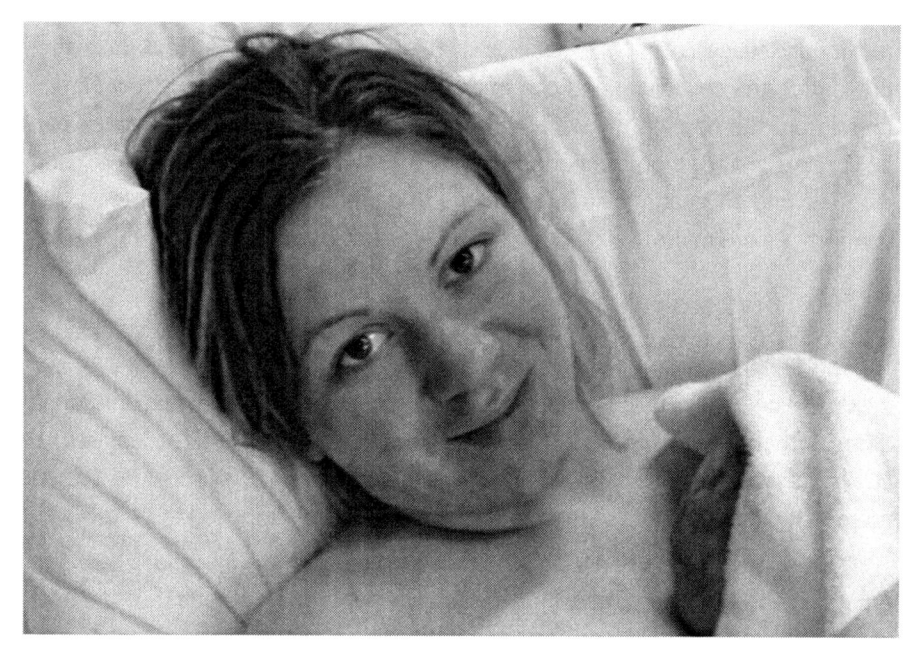

Delivering care from a basic model of meaningfulness will become easier as you gain increasing satisfaction from this more inspirational approaches to care

According to Robbins, it is thinking about a decision that takes time

Frankl (2004) argues that 'man's search for meaning' is the highest internal driver. We know from the Mid Staffordshire Inquiry (Francis, 2010), and many disaster reports (Haddon-Cave, 2009) before then, that high standards are not really driven by monitoring and checking processes but by professional integrity navigated by individual and shared core values. It seems crazy not to mobilise the highest internal driver present in all of us to deliver the highest standards of care to women and babies, and very foolish not to at least try to see if investment in exploring the 'inside' could have an impact. A word of warning though: this will take time as there is no quick fix. It has taken time to get where we are and it will take time to change.

The next stage to establishing core values is to ingrain these in your organisation by identifying the key themes common across disciplines and staff. My experience of this so far indicates that across over 100 midwives in one unit, the key themes which have emerged from attempting to inspire midwives to re-engage them with their core values are love, inspiration, caring, fulfilment, success, striving for excellence, the importance of family life, pregnancy and childbirth, and commitment to team work. By using techniques taken from the domain of coaching and personal motivation, core values can be explored and then embedded using multimedia, including music and pictures, and affirmations so as to ensure that emotional as well as intellectual connections are made.

> Explore core values using techniques from coaching and personal motivation, using multimedia and affirmations

Organisationally, these values can then be used to guide and influence different behavioural norms. This might enable you and your colleagues to challenge anybody who is still engaged in a conspiracy of silence, dedicated more to the institution itself than to the women we are supposed to serve.

Considering what Pert (1999) calls a 'bodymind' interplay between emotions and physiology, as we discussed in Chapter 3, it stands that the best way to embed positive core values is by using all the senses, whenever possible. Drawing on lessons from Erikson, the father of modern hypnosis, it is also necessary to have a mechanism for regular exposure to, and repetition of the desired attitudes and behaviours (Rosen, 1991) so that the attitudes and behaviours become ingrained in the subconscious mind and therefore become habitual. It is estimated that it takes between 90 to 120 days of reinforcement of a behaviour to make a habit, and much longer to break one. If we can build good habits by changing attitudes and belief systems, it is also true that any new behaviours will reflect these new attitudes and belief systems.

In order to accomplish these changes we are going to need champions who are willing to speak out and try different ideas. The first port of call is to get as many people as possible to see that a different reality is possible. However, by nurturing just one or two early followers, it is possible to start the beginning of a powerful movement for positive change. If we get this right, we could end up with strong people who will help us navigate to a new world full of richness, compassion and safety in its absolute widest sense, which encompasses physical, emotional, psychological and spiritual well-being.

> In order to accomplish change we are going to need champions who are willing to speak out and try different ideas

THE SPA EXPERIENCE AND THE FIVE SENSES

As the Pulitzer prize-winning American writer and poet Carl Sandburg (1878-1967) said, "Nothing happens unless first a dream." In many maternity units today, it is as if we seem to be stuck in a paradox of over-stimulation of the senses while at the same time devaluing the senses and the effect they can have on positivity and well-being. As already discussed in earlier chapters, in many labour ward rooms the amount of equipment on show implies the dominance of clinicians and medical priorities in the birth environment. Beds are laid bare with stark, white linen and with incontinence pads which are more appropriate for aging and incapacitated people rather than for young women embarking on a journey of discovery and about to go through a rite of passage.

Contrast these environments with that of a modern spa. Spas make every effort to encourage people to relax—that is their business, their 'raison d'être'. There are a lot of maternity services that could learn from the spa experience. For instance, although spa treatments such as facials, manicures and scalp massages are luxurious, many of them are also remarkably intimate in many ways. Think of all-over body massage, body exfoliation, mud bathing, body waxing and colonic irrigation, to name just a few.

However, within a spa environment, privacy and dignity are taken extraordinarily seriously as people would not return if they felt over-exposed and vulnerable. One argument might be that women using spas are healthy and well and in pursuit of well-being and that the spa experience cannot be compared with childbirth. However, I would counter that most women are enjoying a 'manifestation of health' in having a baby (Winterton, 1991). Despite this, childbirth has become a process that we have deemed to be clinically dangerous with our constant focus on what might go wrong. In preparing for complications and obstetric emergencies, we have done very little to focus on what we could do in this environment to make it go well. Spas are usually painted in rich colours with dimmed lighting. I have worked in and seen numerous maternity units and I have yet to see this philosophy transposed into a maternity unit. There is no reason why colour and comfort could not be incorporated into maternity units for very little money. Many of them already have dimmer light facilities and when there is a problem, it is easy to override and turn the lights on. Equipment can be hidden behind cupboards and furnishings. Sadly, the reality is that even when these possibilities exist, rooms in maternity units are not usually prepared in this manner.

Healthcare professionals are very familiar with the clinical equipment they use daily—so much so, in fact, that they prefer to have it close at hand and on show, than hidden away. Perhaps they somehow find this more comforting, just as Nina Raine found equipment reassuring in the midst of sickness and suffering, as discussed in Chapter 9. In any case, healthcare professionals have seen the equipment so often in their environment that they really no longer 'see' it for what it is. In our busy lives it is also faster and easier to have equipment readily available, rather than taking the trouble to hide it away.

Indeed, under our current philosophy, it may seem petty to challenge every pile of vomit bowls left on window sills or on lockers, or to remark on the metal trolleys on display in labour rooms, or to complain about beds which have lithotomy poles showing underneath. Many healthcare workers think it does not really matter anyway in our current culture. However, imagine for a moment entering a room as a labouring woman or even as a woman who has just given birth and finding it decorated in rich, darker colours like a bedroom might be—so that the colours and furnishings allude to relaxation and sensual pleasure... This does not need to be an overtly sexual environment but it could well be helpful if it is a sensual one. Although sex is obviously linked to childbirth—and there are many reports of some women experiencing childbirth as a sexual experience—the emphasis could be on delighting the senses so as to aid relaxation.

These rooms could have relaxing music being played on entry, similar to that played in a spa. Just having the music to start with gives the message that all is calm because music is relaxing and using it to relax is normal. Women could always stop the music or change it if they wish. Setting the scene with music, you can provide options for the couple to change it or explore different types of music, with silence being a choice too. Remember, though, that silence in a labour ward is anything but silent, as the rooms are seldom soundproofed and labour wards are usually busy places. Women and their partners are likely to find it much more difficult to try and create an individual relaxing ambience when there are no cues to help them when they are nervous, uncertain and, in the case of a woman in labour, intermittently in pain. Soft lights, rich colours, closed blinds, soft music and hidden clinical equipment.... none of these would compromise infection control, clinical care or would cost too much money. However, they might make a difference to women's experiences.

By likening a labour ward to a spa, we may also trigger caregiver behaviours which really protect privacy and dignity just like in a spa, where every encroachment into personal territory, especially intimate space, is carefully negotiated. It is up to the healthcare professionals to set this different scene. In midwifery-led birth centres, this transition may be easier, but it is not beyond what is possible for labour wards too, if there is a professional will to change.

So far we have taken care of two of the senses: sight and sound. Often, in health care, we stop there, even when we are trying to aspire to well-being. There are usually many reasons why we cannot use some of the other senses to build relaxation, confidence and well-being. But why not set these reasons aside for a moment and explore some other possibilities? Another important sense is smell and yet the use of electric aromatherapy lamps has been slow in uptake. It may be that we still lack the knowledge on how little or how much essence to use in these burners and some staff have reported feeling overpowered by them. Yet spa staff who are also exposed to them all day, day after day, do not seem to suffer the same problems to the same extent. I suggest that too little thought and a sense of this being a low priority is behind any inertia to change this aspect of the maternity-unit environment. Furthermore, although the sense of smell may initially seem insignificant, we need to recognise that it is indeed important because during labour many smells usually negatively associated with the body are inevitably experienced—more so during the late first stage and the second stage of labour. These smells may include urine and faeces, both of which are smells that women are usually very embarrassed about. If women are still embarrassed about their loss of control of these bodily functions after the birth of their baby, smelling them can have a profound impact and lower self-esteem, at a time when women need to be at their most confident.

For healthcare workers, once again, this is not usually a problem because familiarity with the process of childbirth enables them to be desensitised to both the smells themselves and also to their potential impact on women and their partners. Using some form of ambient smell may seem an idiotic menial suggestion or a luxury the NHS cannot afford but in reality it is affordable, easily accomplished, and possibly of huge benefit. However, it would have to be highly controllable as some women do have a heightened sense of smell and/or nausea during labour.

The last sense is that of touch. Touch is vastly underrated in its impact on well-being. Caroline Flint, many years ago, suggested that midwives needed to spoil themselves and make themselves feel special by wearing silk underwear (Flint, 1991). Whilst this is usually a cause for some mirth amongst many who have read her book *Sensitive Midwifery,* the point I think she was trying to make may have been lost. Touch plays an extremely important role in relaxation. The skin is an organ which covers the whole of our bodies and as such is the largest organ. We know through the work of Candace Pert (1999) that stimulus is taken in from all the senses and that this then affects hormonal release and physical reactions within the body.

Despite this, in some units we still encourage women to wear hospital gowns in labour. These are modified operating gowns, which can open easily, are usually made of cotton which has been boiled and often badly ironed until bereft of any element of comfort, style or femininity. It is the same gown you would wear for having an appendectomy or amputation. No special thought is given to how women feel about themselves in labour, and what effect it might have. Interestingly these gowns are also usually used in maternity units which, at least, at first encourage women to wear their own clothes… They are brought out as soon as a woman chooses an epidural or as soon as there is a suspicion that complications may be occurring.

This is an interesting phenomenon because many women's chosen birth attire is usually perfectly acceptable for all the procedures to be managed and, in fact, they would not be considered a problem in a real emergency. Therefore, asking the woman to put on a gown could be seen as a subtle but definite physical manifestation of the healthcare professional's escalation to medicalisation. It may be a way in which caregivers feel they can exert some control over the woman subconsciously and enable depersonalisation so that they can more easily deal with the intricacies and emotions of a more complicated birth. Request for the change of clothing usually takes the form of the anaesthetist needing to have the woman's back exposed for an epidural, when it is perfectly possible to fix the back of whatever the woman is wearing so that it does not fall down. Once again, what message is our lack of attention to detail conveying to the labouring woman?

To go back to our spa analogy, spas are almost universally famous for their immaculately white, fluffy and soft dressing gowns, which clients wrap themselves up in so as to be cosseted. It's interesting to note in this respect that cosseting is close to nurturing. Another friend of mine recently had a surgical procedure in a hospital in New York. She has strong, fond memories of being constantly offered 'warm' blankets after the surgery. These blankets, which were kept in warming cabinets, were offered to people in a way to nurture and soothe them as much as to keep them warm. The contrast between this caregiver behaviour and that of midwives or nurses working within a maternity unit, who can only offer rough cold operating gowns, is stark. It emphasises the difference between practical and functional clothing which is based on an ideology of physical safety, and that of clothing—which also serves practical and functional purposes—which is provided to help people relax and give them a sense of well-being. I am arguing that for maternity care we need both.

Staying on the subject of skin, it is important to realise that many women use massage in labour. Massage can bring a couple together and give the partner a clear role in offering positive support to the woman. Postnatal massage can also help women relax when they are tired or anxious and also make them feel special. Within the NHS, we do often provide information on the benefits of using massage to aid relaxation, although use of aroma is not usually discussed. In fact many women and their partners have practised massage. Nevertheless, massage is not included in any great depth in midwifery training programmes, although many midwives teach basic massage techniques in labour and in antenatal classes.

Another issue is that although women are encouraged to bring in their own massage oils, if they want to, hospitals very rarely provide any oils to aid relaxation through massage, even though they are relatively cheap. This fences the massage within a paradigm of 'not normally provided care' and so many women do not explore this option, mainly because they do what is expected of them. It may simply not cross the mind of some women that massage is an option but if it were seen as one, a small proportion of them might not be able to afford it. By providing oils for massage in birth rooms, partners would know that this was considered 'normal' and they might therefore feel more confident to use it. (Anyone with a sensitivity to oils should be encouraged to bring their own.) If massage were really mainstreamed from early pregnancy onwards, through intrapartum care and even on to postnatal care, this would convey the message that childbirth is an intimate and special experience and it would also help couples to cement their relationship after childbirth.

Baby massage is another aspect of massage which could be taught routinely postnatally. Baby massage helps establish a strong bond between the baby and his or her mother and also with the father. It is enjoyable and relaxes the baby. Currently, baby massage is usually taught privately and once again more socially disadvantaged women cannot afford it. Within the NHS, midwives and maternity support workers could be trained to teach baby massage.

The last but not the least of the senses is the sense of taste—the gustatory sense. Smell is relevant here too as both taste and smell are uniquely intertwined in this sense which relates to food, drink and flavour. This is a much neglected aspect of everyday life in maternity care. Despite evidence to the contrary (NICE, 2008) many healthcare professionals still encourage women not to eat and drink in labour even when there are no complications or opiate drugs used. Women are left to bring in their own food for labour. Inevitably this means that labouring women are reliant on cold snacks and bottled drinks. Although some women feel nauseous and do not want to eat, and many others do not want to eat as labour advances, the choices available in a modern labour ward are usually few. Often tea and toast are the sole things on offer and drinks are increasingly presented in polystyrene cups. For women with a heightened sense of smell, these cups are a deterrent to drinking anything, even water. Not only does the polystyrene make the water seem mundane, it is also usually served warm. In a spa, water is served as if it were the elixir of life, which it is of course. Even if plastic cups are used, attention is paid to the type of cup and how it is served. Once again, a small change in presentation could change the emphasis from mundane to special, for very little investment. With a little recognition of the need to engage all the senses we could easily maximise women's sense of well-being and confidence while still delivering high quality maternity care, not only in special units, but as part of mainstream care.

For clinical reasons too, we as midwives must fully engage all our senses to get a wide, clinical, social and emotional picture so as to be able to deliver the best possible care for women. This will involve looking, listening, touching, smelling and sharing food or drinks with the people in our care. Doing this will not only allow us to develop a closer rapport with women and their families, it will also help us to recognise the manifestations of the progress of labour faster and, at the same time, will make us alert to any sign that all is not well.

ENGAGING WOMEN

The next stage is to link with women to inspire them to want a different approach to their care. Many women are accepting of maternity care, with the vast majority of them, over 90% in fact, being happy with the care they receive (CQC, 2010). Maternity care in England and Wales is also now the safest it has ever been (Centre for Maternal and Child Health Enquiries (CMACE), 2011). However, there have been questions raised about the way in which women are treated overall in maternity care, with postnatal care coming under particular criticism (Healthcare Commission 2007, CQC 2010). So although maternity care is good in the UK, I think women deserve better. Women's acceptance of maternity care as it is, allied to our celebrity culture embracing medicalisation through caesarean section on request, is possibly hindering further change, to a large extent. The Maternity Service Liaison Committees can help with monitoring of maternity service provision (DH, 2006) but if we are to involve users we must actively seek to recruit from different age groups and social backgrounds, which reflect the wider population who use maternity units.

Women have traditionally relied on their mothers' birth experiences to advise and support them during their own childbirth experiences. However, now we have at least two generations of women who have had a largely medical model of care inflicted on them so women's traditional reliance on their own coping abilities to get through labour is all but lost. In Britain today there is also a distorted view of what childbirth is like. As a result we now need to look to the new generation of women and colleagues (i.e. other midwives) to help us change for the better. Maybe through Facebook, Twitter and other social networking sites we can spread the word and communicate our wish for a less conspiratorial and more inspirational maternity service that aspires to deliver high quality maternity care in a 'well-being' model, with access to the best medical care when needed. The maternity care pathway must be a social one throughout, but also one which ensures that medical care is given where appropriate.

Midwives may need to learn new skills, accept different hierarchies, build new alliances and learn from the health and well-being business sectors. They may also need to embrace new methods of providing care. For example, there is growing evidence that touch and massage are beneficial to women's well-being in pregnancy and labour. Hypnotherapy for pain relief in labour has been shown to be of benefit although it is still not recommended in the NICE guidelines for care in labour (2008). Neuro-linguistic programming, visualisation and positive affirmations may also all be able to help us provide more effective care. For those women who do not enjoy massage, it is possible that other relaxation therapies involving gentle touch, such as Reiki, could also be of some benefit, especially in the antenatal and postnatal periods.

With these and other new ways of practising, we need to build nurturing into our model of safe maternity care, meaning that as well as providing a safety net, should problems arise, we are also prepared and able to nurture women as they give birth to their babies. Most importantly, perhaps, we need to develop a belief in women about their ability to give birth, and we need to remember that labour can be safe and positively satisfying, as well as life enhancing.

The next chapter will explore this new model for care further, which will involve *really* 'welcoming baby'.

Exercises

1. This chapter opens with the quote 'The best the timid can do is be unnoticed. Criticism comes to those who stand out.' How does that make you feel? Write down five words which summarise the ideas you think this quote is intended to convey.

2. Write down what you understand to be the difference between aspiration and reality.

3. Now reflect on the NASA moon mission… It started as an aspiration and became a reality. What made that happen? Write down five key things we could learn from NASA so as to transform aspiration into reality in maternity services.

4. Birth is described as a metamorphosis—the classic metaphor for this being a butterfly. Think of another metaphor which could be equally appropriate to accentuate meaning in childbirth.

5. The 'spa experience' is used to suggest a cosseting and nurturing atmosphere. Think of an experience you really enjoy and consider how it could become a nurturing element of care for women and their families around the time of childbirth. Commit to talking or writing about this so that, together, you can create a wealth of ideas for new ways of providing care.

Further reading

Centre for Maternal and Child Enquiries, 2011. Saving Mothers' Lives: Reviewing maternal deaths to make motherhood safer: 2006-2008. The eighth report of the Confidential Enquiries into maternal deaths in the United Kingdom, February. Available at www.cemach.org.uk

Godin S, 2005. *Purple Cow: Transform your business by being remarkable*. Penguin Books.

References

Care Quality Commission, 2010. Care Quality Commission Survey into Maternity Services, December. Website: www.cqc.org.uk/aboutcqc/howwedoit/involvingpeoplewhouseservices/patientsurveys/maternityservices.cfm

CEMACE, 2011. Saving Mothers' Lives: Reviewing maternal deaths to make motherhood safer: 2006-2008, pp 1-203.

Deming WE, 1992. *The Deming Management Method*. Mercury Business Books.

Department of Health National Guidelines for Maternity services Liasion Committees 2006. Website: www.dh.gov.uk

Flint C, 1991. *Sensitive Midwifery*. Butterworth-Heinemann.

Frankl VE, 2004. *Man's search for meaning: the classic tribute to hope from the Holocaust*. London: Rider.

Haddon-Cave C, 2009. The Nimrod Review An independent review into the broader issues surrounding the loss of the RAF Nimrod MR2 Aircraft XV230 in Afghanistan in 2006. 28 October, London: HMSO.

Healthcare Commission, 2008. *Towards Better Births*. Website: www.cqc.org

Hoggard L, 2005. *How To Be Happy*. London: BBC Books.

Kirkham M, 2004. Informed Choice in Maternity Care. Palgrave Macmillan.

Murphy J, McMahan (ed), 2006. *The Power of Your Subconscious Mind: One of the Most Powerful Self-help Guides Ever Written*. Pocket Books.

National Institute for Health and Clinical Excellence, 2008. Intrapartum Care. Website: www.NICE.org

Pert C, 1999. *Molecules of Emotion: why you feel the way you feel*. Simon and Schuster

Robbins A, 2001. *Awaken the Giant within: How to Take Immediate Control of Your Mental, Emotional, Physical and Financial Life*. Pocket Books.

Rosen S, 1991. *My Voice Will Go With You. The Teaching Tales of Milton Erikson*. London: WW Norton Company.

Winterton Report, 1991. House of Commons Health Select Committee Second Report on the Maternity Services. London: HMSO.

11: Using all aspects of communication to really welcome the baby

"You cannot teach a person something he does not already know; you can only bring what she does know to her awareness."

Galileo Galilei (1564-1642), physicist, mathematician, astronomer and philosopher

NURTURING NATURE

This chapter further develops the model of promoting well-being by maximising the use of all the senses and learning lessons from the spa experience and explains how our philosophy of childbirth has to move from a biomedical approach that focuses on abnormality, to one where midwives take on the role of nurturing nature, with respectful vigilance for safety.

Nurturing nature may seem easy but actually it is very difficult to achieve in a society which values prophylaxis, i.e. 'Just in case' medicine above therapeutic 'Is it necessary?' medicine. The steep rise in caesarean section rates across the developed world has been driven by the 'just-in-case' value system. This has been possible because of the relative wealth and easy access to high tech maternity care in developed countries, which has given the illusion of caesarean section being a 'safer' option than normal birth. As more evidence is emerging about the longer-term effects on the health and well-being of the mother, her baby, subsequent fertility, her baby's siblings, maternal morbidity and mortality and the overall public health of our society, this is finally being questioned. Also, one good thing to come out of the global recession may be that the challenges of delivering high quality health care in this arctic financial climate may be the much needed driver to change this mentality. As the Department of Health white paper, *Equity and Excellence: liberating the NHS* (2010), pointed out, this new outlook has the potential to increase quality of care and indeed allow healthcare providers to do more with the same amount of money.

Returning to our frontline maternity services, one of the first things we need to do is to re-harness our own emotions, as healthcare providers, as well as those of the woman and her family so as to improve maternity services. After all, emotions are contagious. If the woman and her partner are happy and relaxed, it is likely that her healthcare providers will be the same. If healthcare providers are friendly, welcoming and relaxed, they are likely to inspire trust and confidence in the woman and her family. Interestingly, the same applies, with negative emotions such as stress and worry, so it's important not to communicate these to women in our care.

In order to be relaxed, staff working in maternity services need to recognise the importance of the nurturing nature approach, and be comfortable with using this approach alongside traditional, rational, scientific medicine. An example of this would be encouraging women to use immersion in water to help them cope with labour instead of just heading straight for an epidural. However, given that birth pools are still not available in most labour rooms, this is easier said than done. To help women relax, we have managed to make something akin to having a long soak in a bath a pseudo-technical event that in itself creates a barrier to using immersion in water to help women cope in labour. We need to overcome this and other similar barriers so that we can more easily provide a nurturing nature approach.

BUILDING A LIBRARY APPROACH TO CARE

In fact, anything which does no harm and encourages women to relax during labour can be encouraged. Placebo and distraction are powerful allies to help women cope with labour. By placebo I do not mean fooling or tricking women into believing they are getting a form of pain relief when they are not. Rather, I mean placebo as in using the power of the subconscious mind to encourage people to try different things to see if it helps them.

Antenatal preparation must also start to take this approach because labour is an unknown quantity every time and different things will help different women at different times. I once cared for a woman who was determined to have a waterbirth for her first baby. She spent eight hours in the birth pool, feeling not that comfortable and not happy, but she was determined to stay there because she was fixated on having a waterbirth. Eventually, she got so distressed that she got out, felt more relaxed and birthed her baby very quickly. With her second baby, I was lucky enough to care for her again. For this pregnancy she was fixated on not getting in water at all and having her baby across a beanbag as she had done for the birth of her first baby, but this time at home. Her second labour went surprisingly slowly. So I suggested she take a bath to help her relax. Initially, she was uncertain because of her thoughts about her previous experience using water in labour. However, she got in the bath, relaxed and soon afterwards had her baby underwater in the bath. In this way she had the waterbirth she had wanted the first time. I use this example because women and midwives can sometimes set up choices so that they become an aim in themselves, when all they should be is part of a library of options to be tried, returned and re-tried if that's what women want.

An approach of loaning options rather than keeping them, reflects a 'dip-in, dip-out' approach which expands the ability of women and their birth partners to maintain morale in what, after all, is an uncertain event, laden with emotional highs and lows. This needs to happen wherever women choose to have their babies, whether at home, in midwifery-led birth centres or in highly technically equipped labour wards. Choice of place of birth needs to become just that: a *choice* of where the woman chooses to give birth. All too often today 'choice of place of birth' is really a choice of 'type of care'. For many years, people suggested that women should choose home birth, initially because it would mean they would be treated differently—more sensitively—by the system. The time has come to re-analyse this hypothesis and see whether by suggesting that women choose their place of birth based on the model of care, what they might receive is no longer relevant in the 21st century. In suggesting this I am in no way denigrating home births. (In fact, I am a strong supporter of them.) However, if we are to change the way women experience maternity care for the better, it seems absurd to me to be concentrating all effort on the less than 3% of women who currently opt for a home birth in England and Wales (Office for National Statistics, 2010). The 80:20 Parieto principle of maximising effort suggests you should aim for the majority of 80%. What this means in practice is that we should be aiming to provide the quality of care a woman opting for home birth might expect to receive to *all* women, irrespective of where they initially choose to give birth.

It remains likely that the women who choose a home birth will still have a different and more empowering experience. But by improving hospital birth, we may in fact generate a whole new generation who gain the confidence to have a home birth for subsequent babies. Midwifery-led birth centres could provide the catalyst for this transition, although we are so far down the line of reliance on medicalisation that encouraging women to use birth centres is still sometimes difficult. This is so true, in fact, that the modelling of maternity service provision in London suggested that large out-of-hospital birth centres were not economically viable and the risk that women would not use them in large enough numbers made this a step too far to recommend it in 2010. Therefore, it is most likely that the majority of women will continue to give birth in labour wards or small co-located birth centres in hospitals for the foreseeable future.

Therefore, the greatest impact midwifery can have on improving the birth experience for women today may paradoxically be in our hospitals and not in free-standing midwifery-led birth centres or at home births, where we have traditionally concentrated efforts. While not ignoring these other places of birth, it is vital that we focus on hospital birth and change how our hospitals care for women, de-institutionalising wherever possible both co-located midwifery-led birth centres and traditional labour wards.

ENHANCED COMMUNICATION SKILLS & MODALITIES

I believe antenatal preparation should use enhanced communication techniques borrowed from hypnotherapy and neuro-linguistic programming, to understand how best to individualise communication. Antenatal preparation should also involve exploring how these and other approaches can be used to build a strong rapport and help trigger feelings of relaxation and confidence. This will help women and their partners cope with the uncertainty of labour and the adjustment to parenthood in the postnatal period.

In fact, one of the greatest challenges for human beings is how to communicate well. Poor communication is a recurring problem seen throughout complaints, serious incidents and even wider national tragedies, as I discussed in earlier chapters (Haddon-Cave, 2010). Most communication occurs through body language and tone or volume of voice and the use of language contributes only a small part of meaning. Nevertheless, it is important to maximise the use of language as a resource, because, if it is used to maximum benefit, it can help foster stronger and more resilient relationships, which is an essential aspect of supporting women effectively through pregnancy and childbirth.

Communication can be biased by personal modalities, as we shall see. The vast majority of people have one or two dominant modalities, or internal concepts, from which they create maps to navigate the world and communicate. The four principal concepts or modalities are visual, auditory, kinaesthetic and gustatory (as outlined overleaf, on page 143).

The dominant sense with which individuals choose to relate to the world is determined early on in childhood, with some people arguing that this preference is innate. Most people are not consciously aware of the existence of these modalities or even of their own preferences but, once you know what to look for, determining an individual's primary modality is relatively easy.

At present, midwives and other healthcare providers pay little, if any, thought to preferred communication styles within the English-speaking population. Internal modalities are the inner filters through which individuals make sense of their world, and are relatively easy to discover. Although I acknowledge that in areas with very diverse populations and large percentages of non English-speaking people, it would be almost impossible to ascertain modality preferences. However, for people who speak English, the determination of their preferred modalities could maximise communication, especially early on in the therapeutic relationship, during later stress, or when normal communication patterns are interrupted, such as in advanced labour. By understanding the other modalities, you can expand and enhance your communication styles to ensure you maximise your communication skill set. Most gifted speakers use all the modalities, especially in the opening of their speeches, so as to engage the widest audience possible.

WHY IS RECOGNISING MODALITIES IMPORTANT?

Healthcare providers must be able to maximise communication especially during labour and the postnatal period, when pain, anxiety and changing body image may either directly interrupt communication or indirectly disrupt it through distraction, tiredness or stress. Direct interruptions include times when, for one reason or other, the senses are not being fully used to communicate. For instance, many women in labour close their eyes and so will not be receiving visual signals. In addition, and because of heightened sensations in their body, including pain, women may have more difficulty reading body language. In addition, if they are stressed, their perceptions and thinking will become narrowed so exploring options and making decisions will be more difficult for them. By identifying and using their preferred type of communication, rapport will be established more quickly and maintained and so that trust and confidence in both carers and the cared for will increase.

A sample of interchangeable language to highlight modality preferences

Modality	Example of types of descriptive language used	Emphasis	Communication examples to encourage relaxation using the preferred modality
Visual visual imagery used	I see what you mean. That looks good to me. That's easy on the eye.	Colours, lightness, pictures, images.	Picture a bright light streaming into your body from the top of your head, like a wave, beginning to flow through your body.
Auditory sound and listening imagery used	I like the sound of that. I hear what you mean. That resonates with me. Sounds good to me.	Sound, rhythm, beat, resonance, tone, volume	Listen to your breath. Hear the relaxing, slow, soft rhythm as it resonates through your body, pulsing with gentle relaxation…
Kinaesthetic feeling, movement, activity orientated imagery used	Feels good to me. I can handle it. I am touched by.	Movement, objects, devices, feelings, body links, activity, sport.	Imagine the feeling of a feather lightly touching your head, carrying a feeling of deep relaxation, making your body feel heavier… heavier… heavier
Gustatory eating, food, smell, digestive imagery used	He smells so good you could eat him. A recipe for success. Get a flavour for it.	Taste, flavour, aromas, food, eat	This is your own special recipe for relaxation. Notice the sweet smell of the breath as it enters your nose… Experience the delicious sensation as it travels through your body, carrying a feeling of deep relaxation with its subtle aroma.

Individual internal preferences or 'modalities' occur at an early stage of development and are evident externally through the chosen use of metaphorical language and behaviours. As I've already pointed out, there are generally considered to be four common internal modalities: visual (relying on sight), auditory (based on hearing), kinaesthetic (related to body movements and touch) and gustatory (linked to eating, taste and smell). It is highly unusual for people to have no preference at all and visual, auditory or kinaesthetic dominance are the most common, with many people having more than one preference.

During normal conversation, people naturally reflect back similar language, to engage each other and build rapport. While this is happening it is important to note that some of the modality preferences exhibited initially could have been influenced by other people's speech preferences, including the health professionals' own preferred pattern. Thus it is important during initial meetings that you, as the healthcare provider, take time to encourage women to express themselves freely in their own language and that you are an 'active listener', creating as safe an environment as possible, and speaking relatively little yourself. Individual personal internal modalities can be identified by the phrases people use, their body language, eye movement, their body movements and speech. (You can take a few notes of the types of descriptive words individual women use to build a map of their preferred communication preferences.) Matching preferred modality in language will help you to build rapid rapport and trust.

In other words, while we are talking to women in our care, we must understand our own preferences for language first, and then understand what subconscious limitations this may put on our ability to communicate with some women. Once you can recognise your own preferences, then you can practise using other modalities to widen your communication repertoire. This will enable you to be more flexible in your use of language in terms of style and content, and will enable you to adapt sensitively and seamlessly to the styles and preferences of the different women you care for and build rapport and a good therapeutic relationship. However, do continue to use all modalities. This is because assessing internal modalities is not an accurate science and is heavily reliant on the subjectivity of the person making the assessment. It is also inevitably influenced by their own mood, preferences, level of knowledge and skill. This is complicated further by the fact that many people do not function within one modality but have a combination of modality preferences, i.e. auditory and visual dominance or visual and kinaesthetic, and the fact that these preferences are distributed in varying ratios in different people.

Practising using all modalities is also important for anyone teaching antenatal preparation classes to ensure that everyone feels engaged.

UNDERSTANDING YOUR COMMUNICATION STYLE

The style of communication you use is also important. Are you aware of your own delivery style when communicating? Is so, would you say you are you more permissive or more authoritarian? Do you prefer a distinctive delivery style? Do you personally prefer a 'maternal permissive' or 'paternal authoritarian' style, otherwise seen as an 'invitation' versus 'command' style of communication (Heap and Dryden, 1991, p.6)? Try and reflect on your recent conversations with women and their families. Which do you tend to use most?

The extreme end of authoritarian style is seen in the military and police force where people are indoctrinated into giving and receiving orders through strong, hierarchical command structures. An overly strong permissive style may be seen as laissez-faire and arguably 'weak' in some instances, particularly if a person prefers a more authoritarian approach.

However, there is an enormous danger associated with using an overly authoritarian approach in maternity care because it can mean the healthcare providers come across as controlling and impersonal. A woman and her family with a strong identification with autonomy and personal choice are likely to reject an authoritarian style as being controlling and possibly even unkind, even if it was not intended in that way.

Whichever style of communication is used, using an inappropriate style can jeopardise a therapeutic relationship. As a manager of maternity services who deals with complaints from women, I am increasingly interested in whether it is the style of communication rather than content which has caused the most unnecessary distress to women—because I have found that styles of communication are often to blame. It is often not what you say, but how you say it.

If we wish to give women the best possible care and experience, one which leaves them empowered and feeling confident, midwives must be able to understand the impact that their own personal preferred delivery style can have on their ability to communicate well. They also need to develop skills to be able to recognise when a delivery style is not working, and then adapt accordingly. There may be times in an emergency when a more direct authoritarian type communication style is appropriate. However, when the focus is on choice and individual autonomy, the most appropriate delivery style would be permissive. Permissive styles 'invite' women to consider options and choose whether to follow suggestions or not.

Indirect suggestions are very powerful

Interestingly, the use of indirect suggestions, ones in which the direct suggestion is embedded in language of invitation such as 'You might like to get in the pool' includes the embedded command 'Get in the pool' and is very powerful. People are more likely to comply with indirect suggestions, even if the indirect suggestion is something they might not normally welcome because, according to Heap and Dryden (1991), they bypass women's conscious critical faculty which might otherwise have dismissed the option. Hence, with practice, you can use communication styles to encourage women to explore options for support in labour that they might have otherwise discounted and thus still keep women feeling empowered. Understanding and using different styles could also protect you from accusations of being uncaring or lacking in compassion.

SCIENTIFIC VS GENERALIST INFORMATIVE STYLES

Another common error of communication can occur between people who have a very scientific background (including doctors and midwives) and people who have no scientific background, because the latter may well have a more generalist approach to communication. People with a scientific background tend to have an incremental approach to delivering information. They slowly build up their ideas or supporting arguments until they come to a final hypothesis on which to make their decision. People without this strong rational emphasis often want the information delivered in the reverse order. They want to know what the hypothesis or final explanation is first so that they can better understand the concept being discussed. They are then ready to receive the more detailed information. Getting this particular style wrong means the rational scientific approach comes across as involving a lack of individualised care and suggests an approach to care which is built on production-line information-giving. Alternatively, if you start talking to a person with a rational, scientific preference using a more general approach, the receiver with this preference may ignore you or become frustrated with what they perceive as unnecessary, vague narrative as they search for hard facts.

Sounding too 'scientific' may give your clients the impression they are not receiving individualised care from you

These conflicting styles can be especially challenging when trying to impart the information necessary for women to make choices at a time of high emotions or urgency. These differing styles also play out sometimes in doctor-to-midwife conversations. As a midwife, it is important to realise when it might be best to communicate in a rational scientific style with medical colleagues and also, where appropriate, be able to translate for women both style and content of medical conversations in a way that is both understandable and acceptable to them. If you are able to slip between both approaches, you will be able to communicate much more easily and inspire confidence in your colleagues and those you care for. Once again, begin by understanding your own natural preference and reflect on whether this has been influenced by your background or professional training; then experiment with the alternative styles. Just as in language modalities, it is likely that a mixture of styles will be most effective overall and that by raising awareness of differences, communication will improve.

FILTERS, PERCEPTION AND MISPERCEPTION

In addition to all the dimensions of communication described above, there is the additional challenge of filtering. Our brains are bombarded by so much information every day that the only way it can manage is to filter it and concentrate on what seems important at the time. Misperception, misjudgement and, indeed, error are rife as we interpret and navigate our way in this highly complex world (Schulz, 2010). Hari (2010) describes our individual perception of life as so narrow and misinformed that it is as if 'we are peering at an entire universe through a drinking straw' and then making our decisions based on this limited view.

Women's filters

Some of the filters that women and healthcare providers face are due to professional and social conditioning. A woman's imagined expectation of the care the healthcare provider will give goes far beyond how many appointments she will receive and where and how she will have her baby. She may already have preconceived ideas of personal interactions, potential tests and indeed relationships that might develop in the process of having a baby. As discussed in earlier chapters, this will be compounded by exposure to information about childbirth throughout her lifetime.

One of the biggest ways of creating new filters and moulding women's perspectives and expectations is antenatal education. This is one reason there is sometimes a dissonance between what is taught, and therefore expected by women who receive antenatal education privately, and their experience of maternity care. Antenatal classes themselves are a vehicle for covertly managing expectations in women and thus creating new filters. Antenatal education classes are often seen as a means for providing neutral information but it is important if you deliver these classes that you are aware of the power of suggestion and that you use them as an opportunity to neutralise potentially negative institutionalised behaviours.

Other filters being applied to childbirth may also be hidden personal perspectives of childbirth which are linked to events in childhood, such as close family members' experiences of pregnancy and childbirth, especially mothers' or sisters'. Depending on their experiences, women in your care may range from having high confidence in their ability to give birth to the other end of the spectrum where they may have a deeply ingrained fear of childbirth, tokophobia. Since for generations there has been medicalisation and productionism in childbirth, as discussed in previous chapters, women's confidence in their ability to give birth has been eroded. It is possible that fear of childbirth pervades women's psyche again as it did in the 19th century and in earlier centuries, despite the fact that it is now safer than ever to have a baby in the UK (CEMACE, 2010).

For many women in the UK, the relationship with a midwife is crucial, because pregnancy and childbirth are so intimately and culturally connected to the role of the midwife. This has even been endorsed by the Department of Health for England and Wales in the statement that 'Every woman needs a midwife, and some need a doctor too' (DH, 2007) and more recently by Midwifery 2020 (Midwifery 2020 UK Programme, 2010). Women having a baby in the UK who originate from some areas of Europe such as Spain or Poland, or the United States, where midwifery is weak, often have an expectation of much more doctor involvement and increased interventions, most notably more ultrasound scans and antenatal vaginal examinations, and they gain reassurance from this. As a result, a woman whose expectation is intervention and medicalisation may feel under-confident in a social model of midwifery. Equally, a woman whose expectation is a social model of care idealised as involving a close relationship with 'her' midwife will feel under-confident and disappointed by lack of continuity of carer and may perceive that care is depersonalised even if the care given was appropriate. Moreover, the filters any healthcare provider has developed over time may mean that he or she struggles to see things from the woman's perspective, particularly in relation to the impact the medicalised environment may have on a woman's experience and to her individual concept or perception of risk.

Creating new filters: antenatal education

Arguably, the fear of childbirth seen today is at least partially a fear of iatrogenic harm. This fear has built up over time and is a result of the emphasis on risks associated with childbirth. Even healthy women coming from families with high confidence in their ability to give birth are indoctrinated into our risk model from their first contact with antenatal care, so nobody is spared. All maternity care providers must work to mitigate against this negative effect of the hidden power of suggestion underlying our maternity risk-assessment culture. It is very possible that the very risk assessments meant to deliver safer care have an unintended consequence of undermining women's confidence in their ability to give birth, and instilling a reliance on medical interventions.

Antenatal screening is now deeply embedded in our maternity services and continues to increase at an alarming rate as technology and rational science advance. The interesting aspect to this is that rational science advances on theories are right until they are disproven. So what we identify as a risk today may not be so tomorrow. This means that getting things wrong underpins all advancement in a perverse way (Schulz, 2010). Indeed, it is possible that the price of scientific advancement is being played out in the lives of women as anxiety and stress increase and their confidence and faith in their ability to give birth is eroded in the context of an increasingly risk-averse culture, which wishes above all to conquer nature.

Nevertheless, what is most interesting is that women tend to do what is expected of them. If healthcare providers' filters mean that they do not recognise this fact, it will not occur to them that women in their care are not really making choices. As a result, the subliminal messages of the healthcare system and the hospital institutions combined with the subconscious behaviour of these healthcare providers will create a deeply depersonalised service. Although this may not be noticeable at the time, it may later trigger feelings of disappointment in women when they emerge from the first throes of motherhood and reflect on what occurred during their childbirth experience. It often takes at least three months for women to start to complain about their birth experiences as, initially, they are just pleased to have survived and to have a healthy baby.

We can have a more nurturing approach to supporting women through childbirth, if we acknowledge the emotional work associated with pregnancy and childbirth and the constant nagging doubts that the inherent uncertainty of pregnancy and birth brings, which is compounded by the risk-averse pressures also at play in our society. A fresh and open approach, which includes awareness of the complexity of communication and the human ability to take in, perceive or misperceive information in both the carer and cared for, might help us to overcome the potential for covert depersonalisation. This approach should remind us to provide real, individualised support, which is free from bland reassurance. The new approach will mean that we focus on understanding women and leading them through the pathway of pregnancy and childbirth, using a complex mixture of knowledge and skill, and paradoxically complex communication techniques which are surprisingly simple to implement, as described above.

UNRESOURCEFUL STATES: PAIN, FEAR, ANXIETY...

Anxiety ripples out of uncertainty like a quake deep below the sea which could, if the circumstances are right, come to nothing more than a slightly larger wave which dissipates on the beach. Alternatively, it could build into a raging tsunami, wreaking devastation on all in its path. Pain, fear and uncertainty are powerful elements which can feed the growing swell if coping mechanisms are not instigated quickly and reinforced regularly. Unresourceful states brought on or worsened by anxiety are the antithesis to coping states and must be avoided if at all possible.

If coping mechanisms are not instigated quickly and reinforced regularly pain, fear and uncertainty can increase rapidly

The ripples of anxiety can start with simple uncertainty, especially in early labour, for example with seemingly simple issues such as when to call the midwife or hospital, when to tell the family or when to go to the hospital or birth centre.

Ripples of anxiety can start with uncertainty, especially in early labour. Never underestimate the importance of the first contact.

When a woman does present at hospital or at a birth centre, the initial greeting, whether by telephone or face-to-face, is all-important in setting the scene of calmness and confidence for women and their families. Especially in busy maternity services, it is this first contact which is underestimated in importance and it often damages, rather than enhances, the woman's confidence simply because emotional states are contagious (Adler, 1994). If the maternity unit is very busy and staff visibly stressed, this will be passed on to the woman, either directly through language or indirectly through body language and through the tone of voice used. If the woman and/or her birth partner is stressed, this can also easily transfer to the healthcare providers themselves, who might inadvertently further reinforce the feelings of stress.

Emotional states are a person's way of being at any one moment and they represent something which is greater than the sum of the various 'components' of the situation. Furthermore, while emotional states are experienced internally, there are also external markers which can be measured from the outside: increased pulse rate, respiration and blood pressure, etc. We often believe that states are caused by outside forces but we 'create' them ourselves by our thinking both in our unconscious mind (which is anything not in our present awareness) and in our conscious mind (which filters information).

To change an emotional state, you need to get yourself into the emotional state you want to demonstrate and then lead others into it. Maximising nonverbal communication is crucial if you are trying to change someone's emotional state. Simply describing the emotional state or talking about it is not sufficient. It is possible to change emotional states by using changes in physiology and thinking, because although thinking follows physiology, thinking can perhaps also guide and lead people back to more resourceful emotional states. Understanding this is crucial to enabling women to cope and stay positive while they are in labour.

Dissipating unresourceful states

People in unresourceful states tend to curl their body downwards and look at the floor or focus on a narrow area; it is as if they have become emotionally shut down. If you watch people carefully, you will be able to see which individuals are beginning to slip into negativity and unresourcefulness. It is easier to lead a woman into a positive emotional state if she has not yet slipped too far into a feeling of unresourcefulness. Therefore, if you notice a woman (or her birth partner) developing unresourceful body language during labour, be prepared to interrupt the behaviour pattern being created and be ready to lead the woman and/or her partner to a more resourceful state. This means being ready to change the tone of your voice or to suggest the woman (or the partner) take up a different activity. An activity which gets the woman standing up and expanding her vision a little at first is usually good. However, this approach should only be used if an unresourceful state is observed. Some women become inwardly focused during labour and they are very much in control. This is also the case when some techniques such as hypnotherapy are used to establish a relaxed state.

Other things to try:

- Encourage the woman to walk, rock or change position
- Use touch or massage to connect with her directly
- Use her name so as to encourage her to widen her gaze and look up at you. Using a woman's name is a powerful, understated tool for enhancing communication.
- If possible, get her to smile at something. Smiling relaxes the facial muscles and lifts the emotions.

Embedding triggers antenatally

To be able to change emotional states rapidly in labour to a more positive state, it is worth borrowing tricks from the field of neuro-linguistic programming. To do this effectively in labour, when the woman is likely to be at her most anxious, it will help if you build triggers antenatally. You can do this by asking her antenatally what type of triggers will most likely help her. For instance, encourage her to pick a word like 'Yes' or a phrase like 'You can do it'—it doesn't matter what she chooses. You then have to make a picture of something positive in the woman's mind. For example, you could get her to visualise how she will feel at the end of labour and how she will look and feel holding her baby. It is important to try and use all of the senses in the visualisation process so encourage her to imagine how her baby might smell or encourage her to see herself kissing her baby's head and to focus on any tastes she might experience. Once all senses are activated in her, the 'feel-good moment', get her to pick a small action such as pressing two fingers together or tapping the back of her hand, so that you can later nonverbally remind her of this visualisation (using the same small action, while she is in labour).

Here is another useful visualisation, which can be practised on a regular basis during pregnancy. Explain to the woman as follows:

> First take a deep breath, stand upright, and smile and note how you feel physically. Now begin by stating your chosen phrase out loud (e.g. "I can do this!"). Later on you can recite this internally, if you prefer. Now stop reciting this phrase and begin reciting it again and again and again, this time while performing your chosen action (e.g. joining two fingers together). Continue doing this for more than 20 times, each time making your positive feelings more intense and vibrant. When you're at home you can use music with a good beat, if you like, because this will help you practise this visualisation and will help you to embed the association between the words and the action in your mind. The action will then act as a 'trigger' for the words, which should instantly release feelings of positivity while you're in labour or giving birth. Doing this visualisation can make you feel resourceful, which will be helpful when you need to continue to cope with the demands of labour; it can also help you to break any unresourceful states of mind you might find yourself in (Adler, 1994).

Using voice cues

The use of voice cues is another way to help women to move to resourceful states. An even voice is usually used when people are making a statement, whereas a voice which rises at the end of a statement indicates a question and a voice which is lowered at the end of a phrase is usually interpreted as being a command. However, beware of becoming overly authoritarian in approach with an overzealous use of the 'command' tone because this could be irritating and be interpreted as being controlling.

Facilitating trance-like states in labour

Trance-like states occur during normal human activity and occur when a person's focus turns to the inner world. If negative, trance states can be exhausting and these can occur during labour if a woman becomes unnecessarily fearful for any reason. Negative trances manifest as worry or persistent anxiety and can be set off by shock, pain or hurt. There is a school of thought that some depressions are related to repeated negative trances (Rosen, 1991; Silvestor, 2006). Therefore, in order to maximise each woman's resourcefulness in the face of the pain and uncertainty of labour, it is important that negative trances are not unwittingly induced and that the positive side of trance, as seen during meditation, relaxation or day dreaming, is released so that the women's coping abilities are enhanced.

> **It is important that negative trances are not unwittingly induced and that the positive side of trance is released so as to help women cope**

To maximise the potential for a positive trance, it is essential to provide good antenatal preparation and to avoid negative language or double negatives. This is because when in a trance state, people only respond to positive suggestions and if you say "You do not feel pain", they will hear "You feel pain." Instead, it is helpful not to refer to the presence of pain at all and get the woman to focus on something else instead. This is probably why many antenatal educators and doulas use alternative words to pain and contractions, often using terms like 'surges', which have no negative connotation.

Encourage women to simply let their mind wander and not concentrate on anything. Tell each woman that if a thought comes into her head, she should simply think "Oh! That's interesting. That's a thought" and just let it go, without ruminating on it. During positive trance states, it is important not to interrupt women with unnecessary talking but to embrace and protect the atmosphere of quietness and to ensure privacy and warmth are present so as to facilitate relaxation. Once a trance state has been broken by either the woman or you, anticipate that it is may become negative and decide whether you need to use any techniques to move the woman back to a more resourceful state of mind.

> **During positive states it is important not to interrupt with unnecessary talking but to embrace and protect quietness and privacy**

In summary, every effort should be made in the antenatal period, from the first contact onwards, to build a woman's confidence in her own body to give birth. The social and emotional aspects of birth need to be entwined with medical care. Care providers need to be aware of their own perspective and use physiology (e.g. changes of position) to change mood, if necessary, and also use movement and distraction when a negative state occurs. Involvement of a female birth partner will also help women to cope with labour. Overall, it is important that women be gently reminded of the sense of achievement associated with having a baby and that they be reminded frequently that they are birthing their baby, and that they are not experiencing pathological pain.

PUSHING IN THE SECOND STAGE

There is rarely, if ever, a need to tell a woman in normal labour without an epidural to 'push'. Yet the parody of midwives and doctors shouting 'push' at women as a form of encouragement is only too real in many labour wards and even some birth centres. Instead, women should be encouraged to follow their own instincts and act on signals according to the sensations in their own body. Urging women to 'push' seems to be more about dealing with caregivers' anxieties than about providing relevant instruction to women. NICE (2008) endorses this view when it advises that "in the second stage, [women] should be guided by their own urge to push. If pushing is ineffective or if requested by the woman, strategies to assist birth can be used, such as support, change of position, emptying of the bladder and encouragement."

In this document there is no mention of instructing women to 'hold your breath and push', otherwise known as the 'valsalva manoeuvre' which, although popular among midwives and doctors, has not been shown to improve outcomes. There is even some evidence that it may be associated with changes in fetal heart rate patterns and lower Apgar scores in the baby (NICE, 2008).

Changing this dynamic in a birth room from one where midwives and doctors direct women, to one where women are encouraged to listen to their bodies, will mean a much quieter atmosphere during birth—and this dynamic is becoming accepted on many labour wards. Furthermore, the lack of direction from midwives and doctors inevitably means that women themselves are in control.

Even so, midwives should be aware that they must still work with the woman, supporting her and creating an 'enabling' environment in which to give birth, facilitating movements she wishes to make and identifying various upright birthing positions, which she might like to try, if she is uncomfortable. However, the emphasis should always be on words of encouragement rather than on imploring women to 'push'.

Midwives should be aware that they must work with the woman, supporting her and creating an 'enabling' environment for birth

REALLY WELCOMING THE BABY

Once the head is born, there is no need to feel for the cord, as discussed in depth in Chapter 7. Once born, the baby should ideally be picked up by the mother or handed gently to her soon after the birth. The baby can then be dried and wrapped and left skin-to-skin with the mother.

The midwife should still observe the baby closely and ensure that his or her airway is patent, that the newborn is breathing, has a good colour, a good heart rate and that he or she is adapting well to life. She (or he) should also use the Harrison's birth impact baby dimensions to evaluate health, love and attachment, mothering and self-esteem, as well as the baby's mood, as outlined in Chapter 3. Paying attention to the overall mood in the birth room is also important so that gentle intervention is possible, using some of the advanced communication skills discussed earlier, should any interaction be negatively impacting on the woman's self-esteem.

At this vulnerable time, immediately following birth, every effort must be made to ensure that the woman feels good about the efforts she has made during labour and about being a very new mother. Reassurance and positive suggestions can have a strong impact at this time because labour is a real rite of passage in a woman's life. It is important that partners and birth partners understand this dynamic and do not, in their eagerness to hold the baby, interrupt the maternal-infant contact too early.

Equally, there should be none of the usual rituals associated with institutionalised care. In other words, no additional people should enter the room unnecessarily; there should be no separation of mother and baby for the purposes of weighing or measuring; and no perineal suturing should be undertaken if it is not immediately required for clinical reasons. The midwife should only observe that blood loss is appropriate.

Every effort should be made to ensure that the new mother can truly welcome her baby, making eye contact and using touch through skin-to-skin contact. Women should also not feel awkward about talking to their new babies in 'motherese'—i.e. the gentle and lyrical style of speaking which mothers spontaneously tend to use to talk to their babies.

There should be none of the usual rituals associated with institutionalised care—no extra people, no mother-baby separation...

After the initial bonding period (of perhaps an hour or two) women should be advised that babies cry in different ways and be encouraged to start tuning in to the vocal and body language cues that their babies provide. Gently mention any positive behaviour you notice in the baby (so as to encourage the mother), for instance, the baby making eye contact or mimicking his or her mother's facial expressions. Also, point out any behaviour which shows the baby recognises his or her mother because this will positively reinforce any bonding which has already occurred. The most important thing to emphasise to the woman is that the baby is hers and that there are no real rules to early parenting, apart from basic principles of keeping the baby safe and warm—and of having fun! Women will naturally want to explore the whole of their baby's body in time and this is a crucial reason not to dress newborns too quickly. All birth rooms should be warm enough to facilitate skin-to-skin contact between mother and baby, without either of them getting cold.

All birth rooms should be warm enough to facilitate skin-to-skin contact between mother and baby, without them getting cold

If the woman and her baby are well and the woman wishes to be left alone with her baby and her partner, this should be facilitated but with easy and rapid access to help, in case it is required. It is important that this is made clear so that the woman does not rapidly start to lose confidence when you suggest she be left on her own with her baby, either with or without her partner present.

Mother-baby skin-to-skin contact at birth gives the mother the best possible opportunity to see, touch and smell her baby at a time when hormone levels are at their highest so as to facilitate bonding. Early contact has been shown to have a crucial role in fostering maternal behaviour in other mammals—and human babies are mammals, after all (Rosenblatt, 1992). During skin-to-skin contact, babies are more content and tend to show fewer signs of emotional distress. If the baby is calm, it is important to point out to the mother the positive effect she has had on her baby. If the baby is not content, the mother should be reassured that the baby will soon settle.

Having the ability to soothe her baby early on, will help the new mother develop positive parenting skills so a very small intervention (such as placing the baby on the woman and drying and then covering the baby, first with the woman's own hands then with a blanket) is a cost-free intervention which should be a key part of every midwife's repertoire. In a welcoming-baby model of care, the baby will always remain in direct contact with the mother preferably, or with another human being, provided of course that the baby is well. In a welcoming-baby model of care, placing babies routinely alone in cots, leaving them on resuscitaires and under heaters within the first few hours after birth is a thing of the past. Early human nurturing and relationship-building with parents, using all the senses—sight, touch, smell and vocalisation—takes priority over institutionally determined routines in a welcoming-baby model of care.

The baby should be warm and draped in soft towels over his mother with easy access to the breast, but breastfeeding need not be rushed. Sometimes the rush to breastfeed results in disturbance of the first few minutes of a baby's life. In an unmedicated birth, the baby will start looking to suckle soon anyway. In more medicalised births, skin-to-skin contact and the smell of breast milk usually stimulates the baby to try and feed.

Finally, in a welcoming-baby model of care the labour room has plenty of soft pillows and warm, soft blankets for both mother and baby.

THE THIRD STAGE AND CORD CLAMPING

The third stage of labour is defined as the stage of labour after the birth of the baby and the complete delivery of the placenta and membranes. At the time of birth, the baby is usually separated from the mother's placenta by clamping and then cutting the cord. In the last 30 years or so, there has even been increasing anxiety to clamp and cut the baby's cord to try and prevent postpartum haemorrhage. This is because early clamping of the cord has been part of the package of 'active management of the third stage of labour', the others being administration of an oxytoxic drug and controlled cord traction. Early cord clamping associated with the active management of labour package has been believed to lead to a reduced risk of bleeding after birth (postpartum haemorrhage). However, the timing of umbilical cord clamping at birth in term-infants has been studied to see what effect it has on the well-being of both mother and baby—and immediate clamping does not appear to be advantageous. A recent Cochrane review (MacDonald et al, 2008) reviewed 11 clinical trials and these showed no significant difference in postpartum haemorrhage rates between early or late cord clamping. This Cochrane review also agreed that there is increasing evidence that by delaying clamping and cord-cutting, babies have a larger circulating blood volume and an increase in iron stores for up to six months after the birth. On the negative side, the studies also suggest there may be an increased risk of jaundice that requires phototherapy for the baby when the cord is cut later on.

This drive towards early active management of labour has in the past led not only to the baby's cord being clamped and cut but also to separating the baby from the mother to dry and wrap him and hand him fully covered back to the mother or even at times her partner, while the midwives continue with active management of the third stage. Active management of the third stage of labour is a good example of how, by striving to undertake safer care in one aspect of labour—prevention of haemorrhage—we have unconsciously compromised other interrelated aspects of birth, as discussed above, including the fostering of a strong maternal infant attachment from the outset.

Even with active management of labour, the cord should not be clamped immediately because later clamping allows the full circulating blood volume to enter the baby's cardiovascular system. Some researchers and practitioners suggest that cord-cutting be delayed until the cord has stopped pulsating, although there is little evidence to suggest exactly the right timeframe. During this time, if the woman has opted for or needs active management of the third stage, blood loss should be watched carefully and, if thought excessive, the baby's cord should be clamped and cut and the mother given oxytocics so that active management of labour can proceed as usual.

Of course, physiological third stage is another possibility, which will not involve disturbance of mother and baby straight after the birth. If the woman does opt for a physiological third stage, the cord is not usually cut until after the expulsion of the placenta and membranes. If, for any reason, the mother wants to be separated from her baby, or the midwife identifies a need to separate the baby from the mother *before* the placenta is delivered in a physiological third stage, the baby's end can be clamped and cut as usual. The maternal end of the cord is then left unclamped mimicking the physiological flow to the baby that would have been there if they had still been together.

SKIN-TO-SKIN CONTACT AT CAESAREAN SECTION

For women undergoing caesarean section, if the mother is awake and both mother and baby are well, skin-to-skin contact in theatre at caesarean birth should also be facilitated, preferably on the operating table, as discussed in

Chapter 7. This is particularly important because it makes the caesarean birth a more participative process for the woman and distracts the mother from the operation, meaning that less analgesic or anaesthetic drugs are needed. Skin-to-skin contact also promotes breastfeeding which is especially important since it is precisely these women who most often need breastfeeding support. In addition, skin-to-skin contact ensures that early opportunities to bond with the baby are exploited to the full. In fact, women having caesarean birth are arguably even more in need of the psychological and physical benefits of skin-to-skin contact soon after birth than women having vaginal births—but in some units they are still the least likely women to be offered it. The introduction of skin-to-skin contact in the operating theatre costs nothing, as it is simply a change in routine, but it has the potential to deliver far-reaching physical and psychosocial health benefits.

Routines should only continue if they are evidence-based

The routines such as weighing and measuring baby should only continue if evidence-based and at an appropriate time following birth, possibly on the postnatal ward for healthy newborn babies. Women can also be transferred to the postnatal ward while still in skin-to-skin contact.

Both parents should also be encouraged to engage in skin-to-skin contact to soothe and get to know their baby, as soon as the initial maternal-infant skin-to-skin contact has finished. After all, the promotion of the baby's attachment to the mother and father or significant others should take centre stage during the first 24 hours after the birth. If this means we have to adapt computer programmes in order to enter the data later, we must find a way to do this. We must move away from the situation where routine computer-input and data collection are prioritised at the expense of the care we give. The newborn baby's contact with his or her new mother and father should always take priority.

TRANSFER OUT OF THE LABOUR WARD

Ideally, most women and babies would be well enough and sufficiently prepared and supported to go home straight from the birth room. However, I acknowledge that this will, for the foreseeable future, be possible only for a small number of women, especially with the low physiological birth rate and high rate of interventions currently taking place.

Therefore, some practical considerations have to be given to women and their families in the early postnatal period. Facilitating a 'significant other' person to stay with the woman and her baby should be a goal of every maternity unit in the UK, should the mother wish this to happen. Many hospitals in the private sector have single rooms and although this would take considerable investment, single rooms for women and babies in all maternity contexts (including NHS ones) would seem the most appropriate form of care for the vast majority of women. If this is not possible, at the very least we need to find ways of enabling the partner to stay, as happens more often in midwifery-led units, if the baby is under 24 hours old. This is important so that the father can also bond with his new baby but also so that the new mother will get some much needed emotional support, physical help and reassurance, as she learns her own unique brand of parenting.

In addition, it should become routine that someone present during labour—or, better still, at the birth of the baby—visits the new mother at least once postnatally so that she will have the chance to discuss the birth and create a positive 'jigsaw' of events in her mind, which she can later understand and relate to. This would not be an emotional debriefing (which would be of questionable benefit and possibly even harmful), but it would be more of a finalisation for the woman of the rite of passage of labour and birth. Better still, the woman should be cared for postnatally by the same midwives who have cared for her antenatally and during labour, i.e. by caregivers she has met before.

In considering these and other aspects of neonatal care, it is vital that midwives take their public health role seriously and ensure that all women have opportunities for social interventions that can promote their own and their babies' health and well-being, as well as that of their wider families. Midwives should be reminded that they are in fact obliged by the professional Code of Conduct (NMC, 2008) to do so. Increasingly, health and biomedical care need to actively incorporate actions to promote feelings of well-being. Indeed, we need to work towards the situation where we midwives take on a life-enhancing role. This will be discussed more in the next and final chapter.

Exercises

1. The library is used as a metaphor to describe how to help support women in labour. How appropriate do you think this is as a metaphor?

2. Another metaphor used is the 'pharmaceutical cocktail' for analgesia. Can you think of any others? In your view, are the metaphors you think of good metaphors and what message do they portray?

   Which other metaphors can you think of, which are used in the field of birth? What messages does each metaphor portray?

3. Write a short descriptive piece describing a recent event (about 500 words). Write nonstop and don't take time to think about grammar or spelling while you write. When you have finished, look through your written words and determine how many times you use each of the modalities discussed: visual, auditory, gustatory or kinaesthetic. For instance, when you want to say 'I understand' do you prefer to write visually descriptive words like 'I see', auditory words such as 'I hear you' or kinaesthetic phrases, such as 'I am touched by that'—or even gustatory expressions, such as 'I can taste it'?

4. Record yourself describing a piece of fruit. Then listen to the recording and note which sense you emphasise most.

5. Sit for a moment and think of examples of when you have experienced different forms of communication yourself and how it made you feel. (Perhaps you witnessed an encounter with someone in authority like a policeman or the military... Or did you have an authoritarian teacher?)

6. With a friend or small group of people explore how they perceive an authoritarian or permissive approach to speech. Did any of you or others you have seen ever experience a breakdown in communication because of style rather than content?

7. Write down the positives and negatives for you of different styles of communication. Note in what circumstances you would find specific styles useful, acceptable or totally unacceptable.

Further reading

Centre for Maternal and Child Enquiries, Feb 2011. Saving Mothers' Lives: Reviewing maternal deaths to make motherhood safer: 2006-2008. The eighth report of the Confidential Enquiries into maternal deaths in the United Kingdom. Available at: www.cemach.org.uk

Midwifery 2020, 2010. Delivering Expectations Midwifery 2020 Programme. Available at: www.midwifery2020.org

Office for National Statistics England 2008-2009. Available at: www.ic.nhs.uk/statistics-and-data-collections/hospital-care/maternity/nhs-maternity-statistics-2008-09

References

Adler H, 2010. *Neurolinguistic programming NLP the new art and science of getting what you want.* London. Piaktus Books. (Originally published in 1994.)

Department of Health, 2007. Making it better for Mother and baby. London HMSO.

Department of Health, 2010. Equity and Excellence, Liberating the NHS. July. Website: www.dh.gov.org

Haddon-Cave C 2009 The Nimrod Review An Independent review into the broader issues surrounding the loss of the RAF Nimrod MR2 Aircraft XV230 in Afghanistan 2006 28 October. London. The stationary Office.

Hari J, 2010. We are wrong about being wrong. *The Independent,* Friday, 13 August.

Heap M, 1991. *Hypnotherapy a Handbook.* Milton Keynes: Open University Press.

McDonald SJ, Middleton P, 2008. Effect of timing of umbilical cord clamping of term infants on maternal and neonatal outcomes. *Cochrane Database of Systematic Reviews,* Issue 2. Art. No. CD004074. DOI:10.1002/14651858.CD004074.pub2.

National Institute for Health and Clinical Excellence, Jun 2008. Evidence-based Intrapartum Care. London: NICE. Website: www.NICE.org.uk

Office for National Statistics England 2008-2009. Website: www.ic.nhs.uk/statistics-and-data-collections/hospital-care/maternity/nhs-maternity-statistics-2008-09

Nursing and Midwifery Council, 2008. The Code: Standards of conduct, performance and ethics for nurses and midwives. Website: www.nmc-uk.org/Nurses-and-midwives/The-code/The-code-in-full/

Rosen S, 1991. *My Voice Will Go With You. Teaching Tales of Milton Erikson.* London: WW Norton Company.

Schulz K, 2010. *Being Wrong: Adventures in the Margin of Error.* London: Portobello Books.

Silvestor T, 2006 (2nd ed). *Wordweaving. Volume 1: The Science of Suggestion.* Cambridge: The Quest Institute.

12: Making a positive experience a life-enhancing one

"Learn from yesterday, live for today, hope for tomorrow."

Albert Einstein (1879-1955), German theoretical physicist

A NEW DEVELOPMENT IN THE CARE WE PROVIDE

The last chapter focused on how we can use communication techniques to help better support women in labour and ended with some ideas of what a welcoming-baby model really looks like. This final chapter considers how we can work together to make childbirth truly life-enhancing for women in our care. The report of the working group Midwifery 2020 (Midwifery 2020, 2010) was published in September 2010. Aptly subtitled 'Delivering Expectations', it outlines how midwifery can influence the health and well-being of our whole communities for generations to come.

The phrase 'delivering expectations' is a welcome departure from language which concentrates on 'managing expectations'. Using the word 'managing' could imply a dumbing down of how we respond to what women and their families might want from maternity services and it suggests that our focus is on maintaining the status quo in the delivery of maternity care—so that it continues as it is, without change. This is not what is implied by the report, which states: 'Women and their partners want a **safe** transition to parenthood and they want the experience to be **positive** and **life-enhancing**. ... **Quality maternity services should be defined by the ability to do both.**" (The emphasis is my own.)

What is crucial to this latest vision from all four countries in the United Kingdom, England, Wales, Scotland and Northern Ireland, is that the report explicitly states that having a baby can and should be not only positive but 'life-enhancing'. So often, medical texts, clinical guidelines, policy documents and healthcare professionals shy away from admitting the potential for birth to be life-enhancing. Seen in a simplistic way the report's use of this word could be an attempt to create a strong public health message to continually deliver a more positive model of care throughout pregnancy and childbirth to women and their families. Interestingly, the time when a woman experiences pregnancy and childbirth is one of the few times people enter the healthcare system because they are well. If they can emerge even healthier and psychologically stronger as mothers, it can only be good for our society.

Having a baby is a special event in a woman's life and in the lives of those who connect most closely with her when she becomes pregnant, be they her partner, brothers, sisters, mother, father or friends. Pregnancy and childbirth are like a wave which laps across generations. Midwives can cast precious pebbles into the water, creating gentle, positive ripples affecting all who are in contact with a particular woman's pregnancy.

Prior to the publication of Midwifery 2020: Delivering Expectations, little was said in mainstream policy about the potential for life enhancement as a result of pregnancy and childbirth and healthcare professionals were, in fact, uncomfortable about mentioning the potential for empowerment. This was because if women did not emerge from childbirth empowered it was felt they would have been given unrealistic expectations. Only now, finally, is it possible to engage in a debate about how we go about maximising women's chances of having a life-enhancing experience during pregnancy and childbirth as we set about 'delivering expectations'.

Pause for thought...

When a close friend of mine discussed this with me she said "You can have a positive experience buying a pair of pants but it is not necessarily a life-enhancing one". Just take a moment to think about what makes the difference between a positive experience and a life-enhancing one.

BETTER PUBLIC HEALTH AS A LEVER FOR CHANGE

Clearly, a positive birth experience is very important and contributes to its being life-enhancing, but there is something subtly and dramatically different between a positive experience and one which is truly life-enhancing. Delivering on the physical public health agenda by encouraging and supporting smoking cessation during pregnancy, both for the woman and significant others in her life, will have a direct positive impact on future health, well-being and finances—but will it be life-enhancing from the woman's point of view? Perhaps it can be a starting point, though. After all, it is well-recognised that women having their first baby are highly motivated to stop smoking during pregnancy (in all social groups). This is one among many cases where motivation for improved health and well-being is accentuated by pregnancy and pregnancy is like a trap-door in these cases, which enables public health messages not only to be heard and listened to by pregnant women, but also deeply understood and responded to by the wider family. Maximising this extraordinary commitment of women and significant others to do the best they can for the unborn and newly-born baby is a significant lever for positive change in the wider community. Since midwives are the cornerstone of maternity care in the UK we are best positioned to facilitate this far-reaching public health improvement.

In fact, in the long term, investment in maternity care has the potential to gain momentum and this investment may start changing our precious NHS into the 'health' service it aspires to be, rather than an 'ill health' search-and-rescue service, which is governed by screening, interventions and an acute hospital-unit focus. Any investment we make in terms of improving public health interventions through the pregnancy for women we care for could also involve significant cost reductions in the NHS so that resources can be better used to deal with the people who will sadly inevitably become sick or have to live with long-term disabilities.

So far I have only encroached on physical well-being, which is the more obvious sign of life enhancement. However, if we go further and consider mental health, the impact, although subtle and at times almost impossible to measure, could have the greatest positive impact on our societies as we get pregnancy and childbirth 'right' for women and their families.

In referring to mental health I do not mean the classic interpretation, which is the absence of a diagnosed mental health problem, such as bipolar disease, depression or even anxiety-driven states. These measures are only a poor proxy for real mental health. I mean mental health as defined by happiness, contentment, good self-esteem, coping abilities and resilience to cope with the challenges of life transitions and the ability to support these same elements in one's own children. After all, although it might be possible to measure obvious life-enhancing changes in physical well-being (for example, numbers of women who have stopped smoking during pregnancy; reduced numbers of women who are classified as obese; increased breastfeeding rates; and perhaps a decrease in numbers of women being treated with depression or even maternal suicide), measuring the softer aspects of well-being (for example, increased confidence and satisfaction with long-term mothering) is much more difficult, but undoubtedly possible.

> We need to measure aspects of well-being, such as increased confidence and satisfaction with long-term mothering

Midwives are already poised and ready to turn the key to bring about this change in focus. All it takes for us to make that extra move is a deeper understanding of the enormous power and influence good midwifery can have on women and families, a commitment from every midwife to try and unleash their full potential and a few twists of the hand of fate to release the energy held within for positive sustainable change in women, families and the communities they live in, now and for generations to come. What is exciting is that once this shift has started it will become self-perpetuating, much like overmedicalisation has been over the last 50 years. Because as soon the tide starts to turn, it will start to gather momentum and pull all relevant elements together, becoming stronger and stronger as it surges forward to bring about a real sea change in the way we provide care.

In today's biomedical world, a 'cure' is a totally successful treatment which helps people overcome disease. Nevertheless, as many people know, almost every medical cure has some unintended side effects, so a 'cure' can sometimes come at a price. Pregnancy itself is very often a condition which is not characterised by disease in any form so it does not necessarily need a cure at all; it is only a minority of women who need appropriate medical care because of complications or underlying ill health. Therefore, for the vast majority of women, the medical curative model is inadequate to meet women's needs if we are aiming for life enhancement. However, if we stretch back into the Latin origins of 'cura' meaning care, concern or attention, it is possible to see how the current use of the word 'cure' came about because of an underlying belief that care, concern and attention were paramount to any cure. The Greek word *iatros* means 'healer' or 'physician' and can be observed in words which describe the different medical specialities such as paediatrics, the healing of children; or psychiatric care, the healing of the mind. 'Iatrogenic' also has the same root and is the word used to describe sickness or harm which is caused by physicians or healers themselves in their endeavours to provide healing or a 'cure'.

*Almost every medical cure has some unintended side effects...
and pregnancy is very often not characterised by disease*

Interestingly, the word 'midwife' is popularly known to mean 'with woman', but there was also a word meaning 'midwife' which is thought to have derived from the Latin word *obstetrix*, which is usually explained as deriving from *obstare*, which means to 'stand opposite to'—but which some people have interpreted as meaning 'to stand by' or 'to stand in front of'. This word—*obstetrix*—later came to be used to describe male midwives when they entered the profession and established a medical presence in the field which then became known as 'obstetrics'. Obstetrics marries the Latin word *obstetrix* with the Latin word *iatria*, which means healer or physician. Both the implied definition of the word 'obstetrician' and the definition of the word 'midwife' (based on their derivation) seem inadequate for our 21st century model of care.

MIDWIVES AS HEALER AND SAGE-FEMME

In fact, we need to integrate our model of care with the Human Givens Framework (Griffin and Tyrell, 2004). After all, midwives must now take on the role of healer in its widest sense and become not only adept at providing appropriate evidence-based medical care and be skilled in obstetric emergencies but also be proficient at interweaving their knowledge with advanced communication skills, advocacy and coaching. Within the paradigm shift to midwife as healer, which means the woman is a 'sage-femme' (French for midwife, literally meaning 'wise woman'), I propose that the Human Givens Model be adopted and integrated into traditional midwifery care to help put a framework around the concept of the modern midwife as healer and sage-femme because this model outlines a woman's intrinsic emotional needs.

It is clear that to be effective healers, midwives will need to be equally competent at delivering traditional midwifery skills as they are at anticipating and alleviating women's unstated anxieties. Doing this requires a complex, holistic, individualised approach to providing midwifery care which enables women and significant others to have access to their own resources, which are dormant in their individual belief systems and abilities—and, most importantly, to maximise their use of these same hitherto untapped resources.

Griffin and Tyrell, (2004: 93-94) state that the emotional needs which need to be met for a sense of overall health and well-being cover six broad areas. These are security, attention, emotional connection to others (so that they are part of a wider community), a sense of status within social groups, a sense of competence and achievement, and a sense of purpose. A brief explanation of how these might affect real life scenarios is provided below.

1 Security

Women need to feel secure. The sense of security to which Griffin and Tyrell refer covers being in 'safe territory' and being in a 'safe environment'. Information assimilation is linked to a sense of control and well-being and it is also part of the fundamental adjustment which needs to take place in the face of any change.

Information is usually perceived in healthcare as being either written or verbal and thus as residing in the conscious mind. However, it is vital for midwives and other healthcare providers to note that information conveyed via the senses is far more powerful. Information perceived nonverbally is rapidly processed by the fast-acting subconscious mind. The subconscious mind rapidly evaluates this sensory information, makes judgements and searches for a 'pattern match' to make sense of the surroundings and establish whether a freeze, flight or fight response is required. This is because the subconscious mind is concerned with survival. All this occurs even before we become conscious of it. Therefore, we must become aware of the information we are providing through the different senses and adapt it if appropriate. Consider for a moment what is communicated in your working environment through sight, especially the birth environments you show pregnant or labouring women. What is communicated through sounds? Consider sounds such as unexpected noises, fetal heart rate machines and other women in labour, as well as the tone and timbre of your own and other caregivers voices. What do you communicate through the way you touch the women in your care? And, lastly, consider how smell and taste can convey powerful negative or positive messages and affect how safe the woman feels.

These sensory information cues and their impact can easily be overlooked in busy clinical environments, especially by staff who work in the environment every day. Once the subconscious has set up a fear response, no amount of rationalisation is going to undo it even if on the surface it appears that all is calm. It is likely the fear will manifest as soon as uncertainty or difficulties arise and exacerbate the woman and her partner's response to events. We therefore have to learn not only to tell women (and their partners) that they are safe during and after childbirth but to help them *feel* safe via their senses. Understanding the power of the senses and tapping into them appropriately could help to influence our clients' sense of safety positively, particularly on the all-important subconscious level.

The information we convey also needs to be considered. Inevitably in life people, to a greater or lesser degree, have to learn to live with uncertainty and this is especially the case during pregnancy, childbirth and parenting. Being able to cope with ambiguity is very important for emotional well-being. It is therefore vital that midwives create a safe environment so that any stress reactions that change might bring are minimised. These stress reactions might include increased anxiety or ill health, among other things. Helping the woman and her significant others to be prepared for change and remain in a positive mindset is essential if we are to provide an appropriate environment of care.

However being able to interpret and understand new information or ideas involves our brains being able to absorb it first. In order for this to be the case, there must be a safe environment where individuals can be relaxed in a receptive and uncritical state. This is one reason why you should never try to reason with an angry person. They are not in an emotional state where they can take in new information. Being highly aroused restricts the ability of the brain to think.

Overall, safety should be interpreted as involving physical, emotional and psychological safety. How does this work in practice? Firstly, during pregnancy both antenatal and medical care needs to be offered and accessed appropriately. This means ensuring that the woman is safe using screening tests to identify domestic violence and mental health issues and ensuring that women have access to the support structures they need so that those who are in unsafe circumstances can be helped. Secondly, during labour and birth it is important to provide territory which feels safe to an individual woman, however she may interpret that personally. (Of course, we need to be aware that different people have very different concepts of safety in this respect.) This means that informed choice must be paramount and that choices provided must be real and accessible, and supported by all care providers. For a significant minority of women, hospital will not feel like a safe place to have a baby. For these women, a home birth or midwifery-led birth centre may be a preferred option. Equally many women will choose hospital birth because of their perception that it is safer. Indeed, for some women it may in fact be a safer place for them to have their baby, especially if there is a medical need or they request epidural anaesthesia. It is important to note that what feels like the 'safe territory' to the woman may not necessarily equate to a definition of 'safe territory' for her partner, family or friends and this may not always be overtly talked about if the midwife does not open this topic up for discussion.

Whatever venue for birth is chosen, the midwife must continue to ensure that the woman feels physically, emotionally and psychologically safe while she is in labour and giving birth. If this key need is not met, there will be no way the woman can access self-actualisation from childbirth because she will be concentrating on other needs being met. If problems do arise, it is important that healthcare providers endeavour to keep them as separate problems or events, so that they do not become part of an individual's core identity. This is particularly important when a woman defines herself in the manner in which she gives birth or is able to care for and protect her baby, or when complications arise which can alter the women's perceptions of her core identity. Individuals whose core identity is challenged are likely to develop very low self-esteem, anxiety or even be prone to mental health issues later on.

Of course, there are other areas of care in which security needs to be considered, but these two areas—antepartum and intrapartum care serve as examples.

2 Attention

Women need to give and receive attention so that they can feel emotionally connected to other people. In fact, attention is like an essential 'nutrient' for well-being. During an interaction in which people are giving and receiving attention, the conscious mind temporarily suspends its conscious critical faculty. While this suspension of critical reasoning makes individuals vulnerable, it is also essential if new information is to be considered. Therefore, the giving and receiving of attention is crucial if we wish to influence people's thinking and emotional attachment.

Midwives should note that by giving attention first, there is likely to be a reciprocal receiving of attention. This provides us with a window of time in which we can make a positive impact on the woman and/or her partner and family. One of the universal laws of communication is that because of the innate human need for attention flatterers are nearly always successful, however excessive the flattery may be. This is played out in the criminal fraternity by con men who often use flattery as a key strategy to get what they want. Viewing flattery in the best possible light, understanding this need can allow us to change the way in which we communicate with women, especially when we are trying to build a woman's self-esteem. In practice this means looking for tangible ways to praise the woman's efforts—remembering that no amount of praise is too much from someone, such as a midwife, who is perceived to be in a position of authority. We should be lavish in our praise of women, their mothering skills and their achievements during pregnancy and birth. Praise and flattery in these contexts may allow us to build a self-esteem in women who are susceptible to low self-esteem, for example first-time mothers.

In fact, for a woman's attention needs to be met, reciprocal relationships are key. Many of the relationships a woman experiences are largely outside our control (e.g. the relationship between the woman and her partner and her wider family and friends). However, the relationship we personally have with any one pregnant women is certainly an area where we can help a woman to meet this basic emotional need; we can ensure that it is a reciprocal relationship which involves an equal relationship. If anything, the power imbalance needs to be weighted towards the woman so that she does not feel indebted to us for our ability to care for her. (It needs to be a relationship which is not based on dependency and which focuses women's energies away from any dependent tendencies.)

In order to achieve this, each woman in our care must be given opportunities to give attention back as well as receive it. We can include the partner and wider family, if appropriate, in discussions around the importance of the balance of receiving and giving attention so as to promote a sense of overall well-being in the pregnant women in our care. We can also provide information so as to reassure the woman. For example, we can explain how newborn babies elicit attention by making eye contact, crying, and we can describe the fascination they have for human faces and their ability to mimic actions. We can also explain how a newborn baby will copy an adult sticking out his or her tongue from a very early age. In providing this information we will be empowering the woman and making it more possible for her to make an emotional connection because this information will allow her to understand how the pattern of newborn behaviour matches the behaviour of his or her parents—all with the objective of making an emotional connection.

The midwife has a particular role in fostering the relationship between the woman and her baby before birth, in the precious few hours around birth and in the immediate postnatal period. Encouraging the woman to recognise that the mother-baby relationship is built on giving and receiving attention will help a bond develop between mother and baby and also build emotional resilience in women as they embark on the beginnings of the lifelong commitment of motherhood. Involving partners and the wider family is also crucial as it builds wider support for caring for the baby.

3 Connection

The need to give and receive attention as described above is linked to some extent on a person's need to be emotionally connected to others and it is through the giving and receiving attention dyad that emotional connections develop.

We can most effectively establish an emotional connection by building a relationship in a continuity of care model of maternity care. If we are emotionally connected, we are more likely to be strong advocates for the women in our care, simply because we will 'care' about them. Conversely, emotional disconnection from others is typified by a cold, detached approach to care and this situation is most likely to be maximised by fragmented care.

4 Community

Women need to feel that they are part of a wider community. In fact, friendship and intimacy are crucial to emotional well-being. Social isolation is not only a cause of mental unease, it can also cause mental ill health and even physical symptoms. By creating communication systems which maximise a sense of community, we can make a real difference. In order to achieve this difference we need to work to enmesh women's birth experiences in the wider social community, building communication bridges and thus relationships with other women, workplaces, children's nurseries and schools. This is one reason why children's centres, if allowed to continue to develop, may have the potential to embed health and social care further in the community. By using mobile communication technology, such as texting or Twitter, we can perhaps also introduce women who are due to have a baby at about the same time, within the same geographical area, with their permission of course.

Many maternity services have disbanded the 'block style' antenatal education classes which foster friendships among those attending, through the provision of regular sessions over time, in favour of more cost-effective 'workshops'. In the workshop model, medical knowledge is valued over the relationship aspects of care so the opportunity for women to build friendships across the wider local community is lost. This could be why the NCT's (National Childbirth Trust's) antenatal classes are so successful; they retain the model of small groups meeting regularly. Many of the women who attend these classes make friendships which last many years or at least the months when they may suddenly find themselves isolated from work colleagues and perhaps family, while they are at home with a small baby and in need of emotional support. The need women have to belong to a community of some kind suggests it is time for midwives and maternity service providers to re-establish antenatal education which has a focus on fostering local community-based friendships for women and their partners. After all, the span of time which incorporates pregnancy, childbirth and early motherhood is a time of great emotional transformation and having this go smoothly is more important than conveying medical messages, especially as the same medical information is readily available to most people via the Internet or in books.

One of the challenges is how to get women who do not see this as a priority in pregnancy to attend these classes. It is possible that children's centres could have a great impact, even if only in the postnatal period, when women are likely to attend with their babies if there are child play areas and forms of health and social support.

Another way to encourage women to become involved with their wider community is by suggesting they help to improve maternity care in their local area, after they have had the experience of using maternity services personally. Midwives can encourage women to get involved by becoming a member of a local maternity services liaison committee, a peer breastfeeding support worker, or by getting involved in local religious groups or any other activity that simply brings women out of the home into a wider social arena. Even routine antenatal checkups can be used to provide women with opportunities to develop friendships if we use these opportunities for community fellowship creatively. Building a community spirit in each individual woman can also help us to give some women a sense of status in their social groupings, which—as we will see—is another human need.

5 Status

Women need to feel a sense of competence and achievement within their community. The satisfaction of a sense of competence and achievement usually comes from overcoming a perceived challenge, either in our daily lives or in what we do, what we create or how we think. Earlier in this book, this has already been discussed in depth in relation to the empowerment that achievement in childbirth can bring. This is because of the awesome nature of birth to transform anyone it touches, but especially because of the overwhelming impact it can have on women and babies. We must therefore learn to master the art of materialising the potential benefits that childbirth can bring.

Everyone working closely with maternity care, from governments to individual healthcare providers, must strive to increase the status of pregnancy and childbirth and emphasise their specialness, uniqueness and potential to change lives. Doing this will be the first step to ensuring that the potential for personal achievement currently hidden within the birth experience in our culture is openly acknowledged and brought out into the open. By using this perspective of the power inherent in every woman's pregnancy as a unique experience, it should be possible to introduce this concept of promoting a sense of competence and achievement in women without undermining them.

It is vital that this is not oversimplified down to a process of defining achievement by a hierarchy of analgesia choices or hard-birth outcomes. In reality, this sense of achievement related to birth will always be a complex, multifaceted concept, which is as unique as the pregnancy itself. Each pregnancy will offer the opportunity to stretch people differently. Therefore, we should always place an emphasis on maximising access to understandable information, helping women with autonomous decision-making by enabling choice and then respecting those choices. Informed choice must be an underlying principle even when in the presence of medical, social or emotional complexity which narrows choices for some women.

We must all avoid undermining a woman's sense of competence and achievement. As explained above, we must use praise and flattery whenever we can, so as to build esteem. In my experience, it is the small comments voiced flippantly that can have the most devastating impact on women's confidence and sense of competence, and on longer-term mental well-being.

6 Meaning and purpose

This is the last item on this list of emotional needs but some have said that the search for meaning and purpose is one of the highest and perhaps the ultimate aim of humanity itself (Frankl, 2004). Clearly, there is potential for meaning and purpose to come out of a pregnancy. At the happy end, often a renewed purpose and meaning emerges in response to a new baby appearing in a woman's life, not only in the mother but also in the father or other significant person close to that baby. Even in the saddest of outcomes, some people can find renewed purpose and meaning, as is recognised by SANDS (the Stillbirth and Neonatal Death charity, www.uk.sands.org), who help parents to find meaning after the sad death of their baby.

In our westernised society, most people get their sense of purpose and meaning from the work they do and so become defined by their job and status. For many women, this opportunity is not available, particularly if they are living in poverty. Women are socially vulnerable in this situation because they are less likely to be working and even if they are employed, they are more likely to be in work of a lower status or be part-time and so earn less. Even if women are working they may still enjoy less status and receive less pay than men for doing work of a similar nature (Fawcett Society, 2010). As a result, many women, especially those living in poverty, may not be able to derive a sense of meaning and purpose from the work that they do. Pregnancy and childbirth can transform how these women feel about themselves and their lives, particularly if they are helped to maximise the potential of childbirth to give them a sense of achievement, meaning and purpose. For some women, this sense of achievement, meaning and purpose may well come naturally as women eagerly redefine themselves as mothers and carers. Others may miss the opportunity to build their self-esteem from mothering.

Successful breastfeeding is an interesting physical manifestation of the emotional sense of meaning and purpose that can be derived from pregnancy and childbirth. Many women report feeling in awe that their body can actually feed their baby. The immediate feedback of a contented baby and the longer term feedback of a baby growing and developing can be very fulfilling. This kind of feedback crosses both paradigms of achievement and satisfaction and of meaning and purpose because during breastfeeding the mother is pivotal to the baby's survival.

Clearly, human beings have what Griffin and Tyrrell (2004) call 'nature's gifts' which make it possible for women to achieve their full potential and sense of well-being. By exercising, stretching and exploiting these gifts, I believe that we as midwives can become healers around childbirth in today's society and restore its sacred position to the very heart of our society.

As midwives, we can restore childbirth to a sacred position in society

USING NATURE'S GIFTS

According to Griffin and Tyrrell (2004: 94) we have various gifts from nature which we need to make use of. Clearly, we need to help pregnant and labouring women and new mothers in our care make best use of all their natural gifts if they are to find true fulfilment in birth. Here are nature's gifts, according to Griffin and Tyrrell:

- ♥ A long-term as well as a short-term memory, which enables us to learn

- ♥ Our gift of imagination, which we can use both to detach ourselves from the emotional impact of events and to focus on problem-solving

- ♥ Our conscious, rational mind, which allows us to explore and ratify our emotional responses, query, evaluate events and plan ahead

Our conscious mind allows us to explore and ratify our emotional responses, query, evaluate events and plan ahead

- ♥ Our innate ability to recognise and use metaphors, which allows rapid learning and adjustment, helps to keep us physically safe and allows us to grow mentally

- ♥ The ability to stand back and reflect on matters in a detached 'observer' way, which can help us understand our unique circumstances beyond learning, conditioning or emotional responses

- ♥ Our dreaming brain, which helps lay down previous learning and also dissipate any emotional stimuli not fully explored during our waking hours

- ♥ Our ability to love, which is a particularly strong human gift

The last gift—the ability to care and be cared for—is fundamental to all good human relationships. Being loved also builds emotional and physical resilience across all age groups. Overall, well-being, not just being alive, means that we need to connect with and be concerned about matters which go beyond our own needs.

FINAL THOUGHTS

Much more attention needs to be paid to the powerful sensory communication channels of the subconscious mind and the effect communication through these channels can have on women and their families during pregnancy and childbirth. In order to effect this change we need to move away from thinking of ourselves as 'midwife-clinician' towards a view which is sees the midwife as 'midwife-healer', who in her midwifery practice delivers holistic, individualised, emotionally focused, enhanced communication—all of which can be summarised by the words care, concern and attention. Seeing yourself as a midwife-healer involves an approach which is definitely achievable, which will not necessarily cost much money. However, it will need commitment from you and other maternity healthcare providers who work alongside you, as well as hard work and a real investment in developing emotional acumen. I hope that after our discussion of the issues at stake you will feel that this investment of effort is worthwhile, not only for the sake of pregnant women, but also for your own sake because it will mean creating a more balanced, more fulfilling working relationship with your colleagues and the women and families in your care.

Before we finish, I would like you to take a moment to revisit the six 'human givens' discussed above. This time, consider them from your own perspective as a midwife or other caregiver, who also has emotional needs which need to be met. Do you feel that your own needs are being met on all levels? If not, what positive changes could be made so that your own needs are met, alongside those of the people in your care?

As I end this book, I hope that this last exercise will demonstrate to you just how worthwhile the role of the midwife is to women and their families and to you yourself. I also hope this book has given you food for thought and convinced you that the role of the midwife is stronger and all the more valuable to society when maternity care is delivered within and through emotionally connected relationships.

We already have one of the safest maternity services in the world. Creating a maternity service focused on improving our overall society's well-being through our personal and cultural experience of pregnancy and childbirth, in a way that meets all our intrinsic human needs, is definitely a win we should all strive for. Let's start today and continue way beyond 2020.

Maslow's hierarchy of needs (Maslow, 1943)

- self-actualisation
- esteem
- love and belonging
- safety and protection
- basic biological and physiological needs

The elements necessary for pregnancy and childbirth to be life-enhancing

Exercises

1. Imagine how would you describe to a friend or colleague the difference between a positive pregnancy and childbirth experience and a life-enhancing one?

'Human Givens' necessary for every individual's life	What this means if you are a midwife-healer or sage-femme
Security—being in 'safe territory'	➡
Attention—the need to give and receive it	➡
Connection—the need to be emotionally connected to others	➡
Community—the need to be part of a wider community	➡
Competence and achievement—the need to feel both	➡
Meaning and purpose—the need for this in every person's life	➡

2. Considering Maslow's hierarchy of needs below, complete the empty triangle, after deciding which elements might need to be in place so as to make the experience of pregnancy and childbirth life-enhancing for women and families.

3. Complete the table of 'Human Givens' below (based on Griffin and Tyrell, 2004), from your own perspective as a midwife. Consider what would be necessary to have your own needs met considering what your role and responsibilities would be as a midwife-healer or 'sage-femme' (wise woman).

    ♥ Memory—to enable us to learn
    ♥ Imagination—for detachment and problem-solving
    ♥ A conscious, rational mind—for exploring and ratifying emotional responses; for querying, evaluating events and planning ahead
    ♥ An ability to use metaphors—for learning, adjustment and safety
    ♥ An ability to reflect—to go beyond learning, conditioning and emotion
    ♥ An ability to dream—to learn and dissipate 'excess' emotional stimuli
    ♥ An ability to love

Ways in which I can use what is available to me (complete each sentence)

Memory	I can remember...
Imagination	I can imagine...
My conscious, rational mind	I can think about/explain/rationalise...
My ability to use metaphors	I can use new metaphors to describe pregnancy and birth, such as...
My ability to reflect	I can reflect when...
My ability to dream	So that I can dream most effectively, I can...
My ability to love	So as to maximise my ability to love, I can...

4 Referring to the summary of Griffin and Tyrrel's 'gifts' below, contemplate which of these 'gifts' are best placed to help us make the powerful changes required so that we as midwives can behave like midwife-healers, rather than midwife-clinicians. Then, on the opposite page complete each sentence in the right-hand column in your own words. Finally, make a clean copy of your list of statements and keep it in a prominent place so as to remind you that you have the power to make a real and sustained difference to other people's lives.

References

Fawcett Society, 2010, online content. See www.fawcettsociety.org.uk for up-to-date information and details of campaigns.

Frankl VE, 2004. *Man's Search For Meaning. The classic tribute to hope from the holocaust*. London: Rider.

Griffin J and Tyrell I, 2004. *Human Givens. A new approach to emotional health and clear thinking*. Chalvington: HG Publications.

Maslow AH, 1943. A Theory of Human Motivation. Psychological Review 50(4) (1943):370-96.

Midwifery 2020. Midwifery 2020: Delivering Expectations. Midwifery 2020 Programme, September 2010. See: www.midwifery2020.org

Index

adaptation 1, 22, 30, 70, 88, 92
adaptation to motherhood **101**
adrenaline 1
agendas, national 10, 11
alienation 27, **42-51**
animals 77, 78, 79, – also see 'hippos', 'goslings' and 'wildebeest'
antenatal care 35, 44, 80, 149
antenatal education and classes, preparation, 80, 92, 115, 118, 133, 139, 141, 144, **148, 149-150, 152-153**, 154, 173, 174
anxiety 3, 8, 79, 81, 102, 103, 104, 106, 109, 112, 113, 142, 149, **150-151**, 152, 153, 158, 166, 168, 170, 171
Apgar scoring **27-30**, 55
Apgar, Virginia 27, 29
architecture, building design, 68, 69, 70
assessment at birth **27-30**
attachment 2, 32, 87, 102, 116, 156, 159, 160, 171
awareness-raising 55, 106, 117, 118, 122, 138, 147
beds 20, 34, 35, 55, 129, 130
belief 26, 66, 71, 79, 118, **122-128**, 136, 167, 168
birth, childbirth 1-12, **13, 14**, 15, 18-21, 24, **25**, 26, **27, 28-35**, 34, 36-38, 40, 41, 45, 46, 48, 49, **52-58**, 60, 61, **62, 64, 65, 66, 69**, 71, **72, 73, 74, 76-88**, 89 - 93, **94-95, 96-106, 108**, 110, **111-121**, 123, **124**, 125, 128, 129, **130-135**, 136, 138, **139-141**, 147, 148, **149-151**, 153, **154-160**, 161, 162, 164-166, 169-179, 181
birth dimensions (Harrison) 30-33
body language 32, 67, 141, 142, 144, 151, 152, 157
bodymind 25, 40, 128
breastfeeding 36, 65, 71, 88, 158, 160, 166, 174, 176
Buddha, Siddhārtha 76
caesarean section 3, 20, 37, 64, 69, 71, 75, **79-85, 88**, 89, 93, 99, 100, 113, 114, 135, 138, **159-160**
Calvino, Italo 52
Care Quality Commission (CQC) 11, 15, **19**, 44, **55**, 65, 96, 97, 135

Cartesian dualism 5, 24, 27, 40
catecholamines 1
Changing Childbirth **5**, 10, 18, **38**
childbirth – see 'birth'
Cinderella service 65, 96-97, 108
clock time 13, 21, 112
co-dependency 1
Commissioning for Quality and Innovation 20
communication 10, 12, 62, **66**, **67**, **138-163**, 164, 168, 171, 173, 178
community 2, 4, 7, 13, 14, 34, 91, 105, 166, 168, 173, 174, 180
complications 3, 69, 80, 81, 85, 113, 129, 132, 134, 167, 171
connection 76, 77, 114, 128, 168, 172, **173**, 180
cord clamping 86, **158**
cord cutting – see 'cutting the cord'
core values 64, 118, 125, **126**, **127**, **128**
culture 4, 7, 8, 11, 20, 21, 24, 43, 46, 53, 57, 58, 59, 65, 67, 71, 84, 90, 91, 118, 125, 126, 130, 135, 149, 175
cure 167
cutting the cord 87, **94**, **158**
decision making, decide 30, 56, 75, 43, 48, 71, 82, 84, 92, 106, 118, **122-123**, 124, **126**, 142, 146-147, 154, 175, 179
delivery 4, 10, 12, 21, **40**, 45, **52-63**, 64-75, 83, 145, 158, 164
delivery suites 52, 57, 59, 61, 64, 65, 67, 68, 69, 71, 72, 73, 74, 75
Deming, William Edwards **42-50**, 125, 137
depersonalisation 4, 12, 37, 55, 57, 61, 65, 72, 73, 85, 116, 132, 149, 150
Descartes 24 – also see 'Cartesian dualism'
disasters 46, 127, 143
Down's Syndrome 44, 101
dualism – see 'Cartesian dualism'
early discharge 105
efficiency 34 - 35, 42,- 50, 74
EFM – see 'electronic fetal monitoring'
Einstein, Albert 164
electronic fetal monitoring (EFM) 37, 80, 81,
emergencies 3, 58, 69, 70, 118, 129, 132, 145, 168

emotion, emotional, 2, 3, 4, 7, 8, 11, 12, 13, 14, **25**, 26, 30-33, 54, 55, 61, 67, 74, **76, 77**, 79, 80, 82, 85, 86, 90, 93, 95, 97, 98, 99, **100**, 101, 104-106, 113, 116, 120, 124-126, 128, 132, 134, 139, 140, 147, 150, 151, **152-154**, 157, 161, 168, 170, **172**, 173-178, 180
emotional resilience 2, 8, 61, 77, 93, 166, 172, 177
emotional support 96, 97, **100**, 101, 161, 174
Emperor's new clothes 52, 61
empower, empowerment 13, 43, 47, 48, 57, 61, 73, 83, 84, 140, 145, 146, 165, 172, 174
epidurals 46, 59, 72, 83, **84**, 86, 100, 113, 115, 116, 119, 132, 139, 155, 170
equipment 48, 68, 70, 89, 112, 114, 115, 116, 123, 124, 129, 130
ethics 40, 98
exercises **8, 21, 40**, 47, **50, 62, 74, 93, 108, 120, 136, 162, 179**
external validation 47, 48, 49
facilitating trance-like states 153
fathers 1, 7, 14, 30, 31, 32, 61, 78, 87, 93, 94, 104, 128, 134, 160, 161, 165, 176
fear 1, 46, 52, 57, 70, 80, 81, 90, 113, 120, 125, 148, 149, 150, 153, 169
feeling 1, 81, 93, 97, **99-105**, 109, 126, 141, 143, 149, 151, 153, 161, 176
fetal blood sampling 55, 79, 82, 86
filters 142, **147-149**, 151
finance 19, 47, 165
first stage 112, 131,
forceps 2, 81, 85, 113
Ford 5, 34, 101
Fordism 34, 35, 38, 42
fragmented care 4, 5, 12, 13, 15, 24, 25, 30, 35, 38, 44, 45, 84, 173
Francis Report (Mid Staffordshire Report) 20, 21, 22, 46, 47, 127
free (services) **18**, 21
Fromm, Erich 96
Galilei, Galileo 138
geese – see 'goslings'
Godin, Seth 122
goslings 77, 93

Hanzak, Elaine 2
Harrison, Michelle 30-33, 156
Harrison's questions 30-33
healer, midwife as 167, **168**, 176, 178, 180
Healthcare Commission 11, **19-20**, 65, 85, 96, 135
Healthcare Commission Enquiry 11
hierarchies 11, 14, 35, 46, 125, 135, 145, 179,
hippopotomi 78
holistic approaches 5, 35, 168, 178,
home birth 14, 34, 37, 48, 49, 93, 118, 140, 141, 170
horoscopes 8
hospital gowns 35, 58, 59, 68, 72, 132, 133
hospitals 3, 4, 14, 15, 18, **19-21**, 34-37, 46, 48, 54, 58, 59, 62, 64, 65, 68,
    70, 71, 72, 81, 82, 84, 89, 91, 93, 96, 97, 100, 103, 104, 105, 108,
    112, 113, 114, 115, 116, 122, 123, 132, 133, 140, 141, 149, 150,
    151, 160, 161, 166, 170
hospital design 62, 71
Human Givens 168, 178, 180, 181
hysterectomy 56, 79, 82
imagery 143
imprinting 14, 76, 77, 79, 80, 81, 93
incontinence pads 58, 68, 129
individualised care 5, 38, 74, 85, 146, 150, 168, 178
industrialisation 21, 34, 35, 37, 38, 40, 47, 80
informative styles 146
insecurity 1
intervention (s) 4, 12, 26, 28, 40, 44, 45, 55, 56, 79, 83, 84, 90, 93, 108,
    109, 113, 114, 115, 116, 148, 149, 156, 157, 161, 166
institutionalisation 2, 11, 12, **14, 15, 18, 19**, 54, 59, 61, 65, 92, 103, 123,
    124, 141, 148, 156, 157, 158
intrapartum 29, 55, 65, 133, 171
intrinsic motivation 47, 49, 50
'just-in-case' mentality 35, 56, 70, 80, 82, 91, 138
Kirkham, Mavis 11, 12, 22, 23, 50, 123, 137
King's Fund 11, 12, 22, 23, 60, 63

labour 3, 5, 12, 15, 18, 25, 30, 32, 33, 35, 36, 37, 38, 40, 46, 49, 52, **53-59,
    61, 62, 64-68**, **70-74**, 78-81, **82-84**, 89, 93, **98, 99, 100**, 101, 103,
    106, **110-116**, 129-136, 139-142, 146, 150-156, 158-162, 164, 169,
    170, 171, 177
language 32, 37, 50, **52-63**, **64, 66, 67, 72, 73, 75**, 89, 94, 97, 141, 142,
    143, 144, 146, 147, 151, 152, 154, 157, 164
language guard 75
layout 68, 70
lean management **42-50**
library approach to care 139-141
life-enhancing care 161, 164-181
litigation 42, 79, 82
Lorenz, Konrad 77
Making It Better for Mother and Baby 10
massage 129, 133, 134, 135, 136, 152
matching set syndrome 68-69
maternal-infant attachment 2, 102, 116
Maternity Matters 10, 38, 49
Mead, Margaret 4
meaning 27, 53, 54, 67, 82, 116, **125-127**, 136, 160, 167, 168, 175, **176**,
    180
[The] Meaning of Life (Monty Python) 116
media 49, 62, 69, 77, 80, 108, **110-121**,
medicalisation 11, 14, 34, 37, 49, 54, 65, 80, 83, 84,103, 114, 116, 124,
    132, 135, 140, 148, 149, 158, 167
medical model of care 21, 53, 135
memory 13, 77, 79, 98, 177, 180, 181
mental health issues 1, 2, 3, 45, 166, 171
metaphors 108, 114, 115, 136, 143, 162, 177, 180, 181
Mid-Staffordshire Foundation Trust 20, 21, 22, 46, 47, 127
midwife-clinicians 178
Midwifery 2020 10, 18, 45, 148, 164, 165
midwifery-led care 12, 45, 46, 48, 49, 50, 115, 131, 140, 141, 170
midwives 10, 11, 12, 18, 19, 29-31, 32, 34, 35 37, 44-48, 50, **52-57**, 59, 60,
    62, 66, 69, 72, 81, **84-89**, 91, 92, 93, 97, 100, 104, 110-116, 118,
    123, 124, 125, 127, 132, 133, 134, 135, 138, 140, 142, 145, 146,
    155, 159, 161, **165-176**, 180,

Midwives Act (1902) 34
modalities 70, **141-144**, 147, 162
model (s) of care 5, 11, 21, 30, 85, 92, 105, 108, 122, 135, 140, 148, 149, 157, 158, 164. 168
Morrison, Jim 110,
motivation, intrinsic 47, 49, 50,
National Childbirth Trust (NCT) 15, 36, 38, 58, 96, 97, 99, 100, 173
National Institute for Health and Clinical Excellence – see 'NICE'
National Service Framework for Children and Young People 10, 38, 49
Nature's Gifts 176-177
NCT – see 'National Childbirth Trust'
neonatal units 71
newspapers 112, 118
NHS Plan 43
NICE 3, 55, 65, 67, 69, 134, 155
Nimrod Review 46, 51, 137, 163
normality, promoting 14, 20, 49, 70, 92, 116, 118
Northwick Park Maternity Hospital 11, 20, 23
nuchal cord 86
nurturing nature 138, 139
Oakley, Ann 37, 65
Odent, Michel 2, 37, 80
oils, massage 133
One Born Every Minute 110, 111, 121
one-to-one care in labour 59
overmedicalisation 37, 167
passenger, baby as 25, 39
patients 60, 61
Peel Report 14, 15, 23, 34
perception 8, 18, 21, 34, 46, 62, 65, 69, 97, 98, 103, 108, 110-121, 147, 149, 170, 171
Pictionary 74
placebos 26, 40, 139
place of birth 14, 115, 140
politics 2, 19, 37, 38, 43, **52-63**, 76
postnatal care 35, 37, 71, 96, 97, 100, 103, 108, 133, 135

power 11, 18, 19, 26, 33, 37, 50, 52, 55, 57, 59, **61-74**, 76, 87, 117, 139,148, 149, 167, 169, 172, 175. 180
powerful, feelings 16, 19, 32, 33,34, 37, 49, 57, 61, 65, 67, 74, 76, 77, 92, 100, 111, 114, 122, 124, 128, 139, 146, 150, 152, 169, 178, 180
preferences, professional 70
production line 5, 31, 34, 35, 37, 40, 52, 125, 146
professional preferences 70
promoting normality 20, 49, 118
protectiveness 102-105
psychological co-dependency 1
psycho-social model of care 11, 21
public health 13, 14, 138, 161, 164, 165
purpose and meaning 7, 14, 80, 133, 168, **175, 176**, 180
pushing 55, 115, 155
quality of care 15, 19, 20, 45, 47, 138, 140
randomised controlled trials (RCTs) 26, 40
reductionist approaches 40
Reiki 136
relationships 2, 8, 10, 12, 13, 30, 44, 45, 61, 110, 141, 147, 172, 173, 177, 178
rescuer-victim modality 70
resourceful states 150-154
rite of passage, birth as a 4, 73, 102, 106, 108, 109, 129, 156, 161
ritualisation **76-95**, 122
Safe Birth: Everybody's Business 22, 23
safety 7, 11, 12, 16, 18, 20, 21, 61, 69, 79, 85, 90, 92, 110, 115, 118, 128, 133, 136, 138, 169, 170, 179, 180
sage-femme, midwife as 168, 180
Saunders, Dame Cicely 13
second stage 55, 69, 83, 84, 115, 131, 155
security 105, 168, **169-171**, 180
Seeing the Person in the Patient 60, 63
self-actualisation 171
senses 122, **128-134**, 138, 142, 152, 158, 169,
Shribman, Sheila 10
skin-to-skin contact 32, 33, 54, 86, 88-90, 92, 94, **156-160**

Sleeping Beauty 10-11
Smith, Lillian 1
Sontag, Susan 42
spa experience 118, 129, 136, 138
status 19, 47, 92, 101, **102**, **104**, 164. 168, **174-176**
student midwives 7, 48, 75
subliminal messages 65, 74, 87, 93, 103, 114, 149
suites, delivery 52, 58, 59, 61, **64-75**
teamwork 11, 72
television (programmes) 11, 72, 110, 113, 114, 118
terminology **52-63**, 65, 72, 73
The Three Ps (powers, passage, passenger) 25, 39
theatre 57, 69, 88, 99, 112, 116, 159, 160
thinking and language 61, 66
third stage 158 -159
touch 31, 32, 89, 122, 124, 132, 135, 136, 152, 156, 157, 158, 169, 175
Toyota 42-43, 46
trance-like states 153
transfer out of the labour ward 160
transition 33, 35, 84, 92, 96, **101-109**
trauma 1
triggers, embedding them antenatally 152
unresourceful states – also see 'resourceful states' **150-153**
utilitarian focused maternity care 4, 5
utilitarianism 4
ultrasound scans 17, 44, 112, 148
validation, external 47-49
values 4, 11, 13, 15, 20, 30, 48, 49, 64, 118, 123 -128, 138
ventouse 2, 56, 81, 83, 113
voice cues 153
Wagner, Marsden 7
weighing the baby 2, 54, 56, 81, 83, 90, 91, 113, 156, 160
wildebeest 78, 94
Winterton Report 10, 38, 129
Wittgenstein, Ludwig 63, 64, 66

Also available...

Books to help your women prepare for a normal birth...

Birth: Countdown to Optimal: information and inspiration for pregnant women—by Sylvie Donna

Birthing Normally After a Caesarean or Two: exploring reasons and practicalities for VBAC—by Hélène Vadeboncoeur

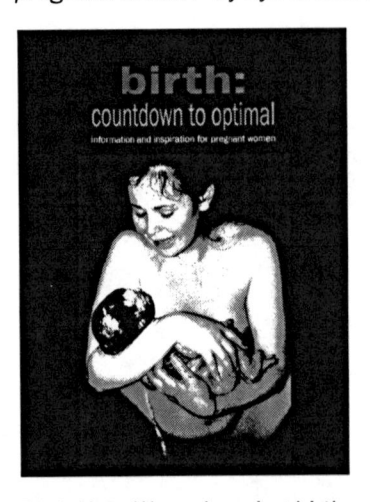

Birth Your Way: choosing birth at home or in a birth centre by Sheila Kitzinger

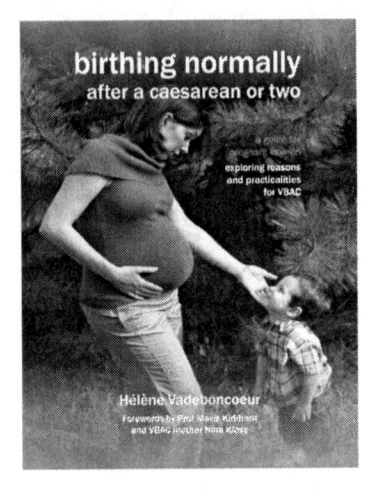

Birth Pain: Power to Transform: a guide for pregnant women—by Verena Schmid

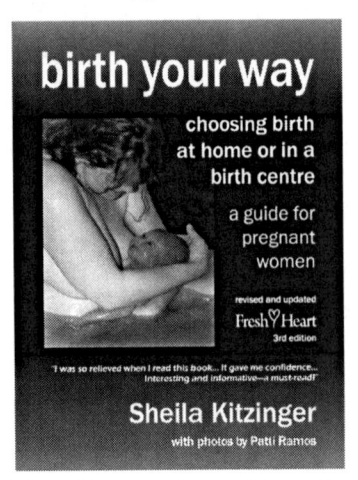

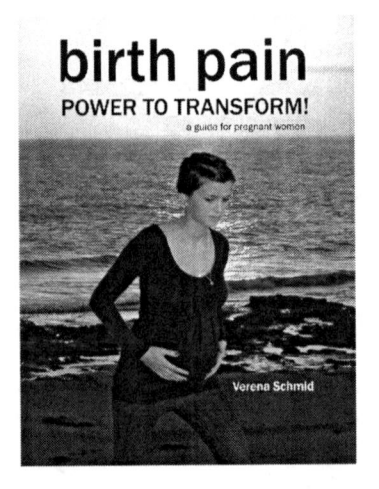

Also available

Books you yourself may find useful...

*Optimal Birth: What, Why & How—
a reflective narrative approach based
on research evidence*—by Sylvie Donna

*Birth Pain: Explaining sensations,
exploring possibilities*—
by Verena Schmid

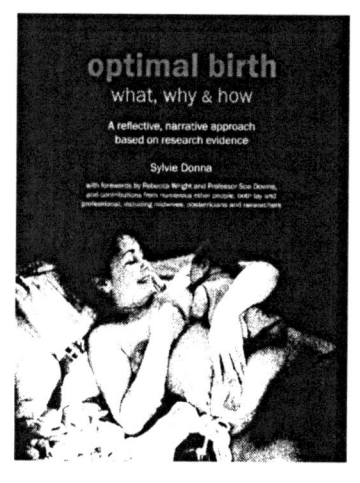

*Surprising, Inspiring Birth: accounts of
birth to inform, amuse and reassure*—
by Sylvie Donna (ed)

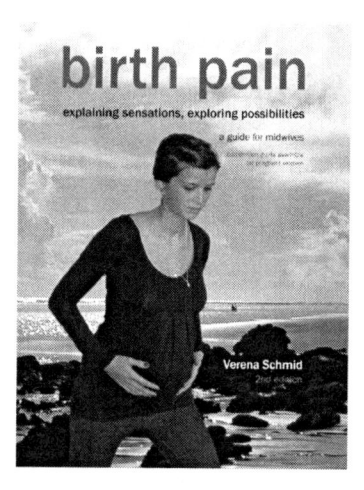

*Promoting Normal Birth: Research,
Reflections & Guidelines*—
an international collaboration

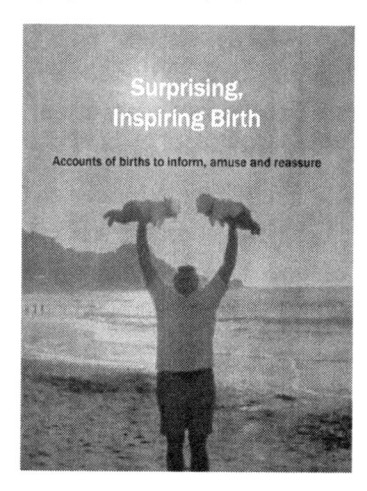

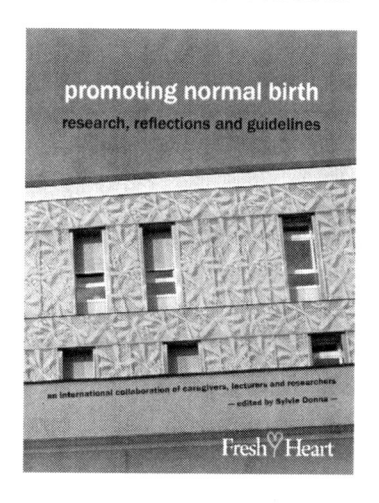

See the website for info and prices. All books are also available from Amazon.

www.freshheartpublishing.co.uk

About the author

Debby Gould initially trained as a midwife, beginning with nursing training, since there were very few direct-entry midwifery courses when she trained. She was inspired to become a midwife by her older sister, Cathy, who had a home birth with her second son. The magic of the celebration of that birth has never left her and although Debby was not allowed to witness the birth she well remembers the positive impact the midwife had on the female members of her family.

As the fifth girl in a family of six, where the boys were always given priority, Debby found it refreshing to see a reversal of the normal paternalistic hierarchy during the home birth. The new mother was treasured and made to feel special and the midwife was also greeted as an important guest.

The magic of the atmosphere around one birth has never left her and it was this that inspired the author to become a midwife

Initially, getting a midwifery post was difficult in Portsmouth in 1984 so Debby took a part-time post in what was then called a GP unit. (It is now known as a co located midwifery-led unit.) This was not Debby's first choice of post, having anticipated consolidating her training in a busy consultant-led unit but it was certainly life-changing. After feeling disillusioned during her training, Debby quickly fell back in love with midwifery and the midwifery profession as she learned to support normal birth and watch women give birth to their babies without interventions. Thus the seeds were sown for Debby's midwifery career, which has involved championing normality and promoting woman-centred care.

Initially, Debby spent 14 years working as a midwife in the Portsmouth area and this included working in a consultant-led unit, a co-located birth centre, a stand-alone birth centre and also working within the community. While she was a community midwife the author attended home births, including some water births at home. It was during this time that Debby gave birth to her own two sons in 1988 and 1989. She also continued studying and obtained a BSc and an MSc (achieving the last with distinction)—as well as becoming a hypnotherapist along the way too. It was as a result of Debby's MSc work that her concept analysis of normal labour was written, which was a seminal piece of work for grounding midwifery in normality. This was published in the *Journal of Advanced Nursing* in 2000.

With a strong grounding in clinical practice and now a Master's degree, Debby left Portsmouth and became the Practice Development Midwife at Guy's and St Thomas' Hospital in London. She then became High Care Manager at Princess Ann Hospital in Southampton, where she had responsibility as a labour ward manager working with high risk women. It was here that Debby met Maggie Elliott, who was later to become Maggie O'Brien and the President of the Royal College of Midwives.

Maggie exposed Debby to the political side of midwifery, which resulted in Debby becoming a Royal College of Midwives (RCM) council member in 2001. Debby later went on to become Deputy Chair of the RCM Council in 2005 and Chair of the RCM from 2007-2011, completing two full terms in office. Debby's career continued to progress: she was Head of Midwifery in Winchester, then became one of the first consultant midwives in the UK at Queen Charlotte's Hospital birth centre in London. Three years later she returned to a Head of Midwifery role when she took up a secondment at St George's Hospital, London and she currently works as Head of Midwifery at University College London Hospitals (UCLH). She is also named in Debrett's *People of Today* as one of the top 25,000 influential and successful people in the UK.

Debby has built a strong reputation for public speaking and political commentary on maternity care. During her time as an RCM council member she helped to launch the Campaign for Normal Birth and her role in promoting normality has continued since then. She is on the advisory faculty for the Advanced Life Support in Obstetrics Course. She has acted as advisor and promoter of normality and this has involved working on Scottish normal birth initiatives, speaking in Abu Dhabi, Poland and Southern Ireland and being a returning speaker to the Royal College of Obstetrician and Gynaecologists Advanced Labour Ward Skills courses. Debby is also a member of the *British Journal of Midwifery* editorial board, and if you wish to know more about her views and ideas you might like to follow her Birth Rite column in the *British Journal of Midwifery*, which she has been writing since 2001.

As this book demonstrates, today Debby is as passionate as ever about giving women high quality maternity care through excellent midwifery. She believes that the pivotal role that midwives and midwifery can contribute to the well-being of our society is both underestimated and under-utilised. This book provides an insight into some of the ways in which she believes midwives can make more of a contribution to the well-being of both mother and babies.

Lightning Source UK Ltd.
Milton Keynes UK
UKOW02f0210101013

218778UK00003B/75/P

9 781906 619169